国家卫生健康委员会住院医师规范化培训规划教材

住院医师英语手册

第2版

主　编　唐熠达

副主编　张　龑　蔡世荣　潘　慧　金泽宁

U0207793

人民卫生出版社

·北　京·

版权所有，侵权必究！

图书在版编目（CIP）数据

住院医师英语手册/唐熠达主编. —2版. —北京：
人民卫生出版社，2022.1（2024.11 重印）
国家卫生健康委员会住院医师规范化培训规划教材
ISBN 978-7-117-32745-9

Ⅰ. ①住… Ⅱ. ①唐… Ⅲ. ①医学－英语－职业培训
－教材 Ⅳ. ①R

中国版本图书馆 CIP 数据核字（2021）第 281600 号

人卫智网	www.ipmph.com	医学教育、学术、考试、健康，
		购书智慧智能综合服务平台
人卫官网	www.pmph.com	人卫官方资讯发布平台

住院医师英语手册
Zhuyuan Yishi Yingyu Shouce
第 2 版

主　　编：唐熠达
出版发行：人民卫生出版社（中继线 010-59780011）
地　　址：北京市朝阳区潘家园南里 19 号
邮　　编：100021
E - mail：pmph @ pmph.com
购书热线：010-59787592　010-59787584　010-65264830
印　　刷：中农印务有限公司
经　　销：新华书店
开　　本：850×1168　1/32　　印张：10.5
字　　数：240 千字
版　　次：2015 年 10 月第 1 版　　2022 年 1 月第 2 版
印　　次：2024 年 11 月第 3 次印刷
标准书号：ISBN 978-7-117-32745-9
定　　价：45.00 元

打击盗版举报电话：010-59787491　E-mail：WQ @ pmph.com
质量问题联系电话：010-59787234　E-mail：zhiliang @ pmph.com

编者名单

编　　委（按字母顺序排序）

蔡世荣　中山大学附属第一医院

金泽宁　首都医科大学附属北京天坛医院

李　萍　中国医学科学院阜外医院

穆　荣　北京大学第三医院

潘　慧　北京协和医院

唐熠达　北京大学第三医院

叶　清　上海交通大学医学院附属仁济医院

张　龑　北京大学第三医院

周芙玲　武汉大学中南医院

Michael X. Yang　University of California

James Shue-Min Yeuh　Imperial College London

数字编委（按字母顺序排序）

毕新刚　中国医学科学院肿瘤医院

程真顺　武汉大学中南医院

李德岭　首都医科大学附属北京天坛医院

隋　准　北京大学人民医院

吴　东　北京协和医院

邢　燕　北京大学第三医院

朱颖华　上海交通大学医学院附属仁济医院

编写秘书　李　萍　中国医学科学院阜外医院

出版说明

　　为配合 2013 年 12 月 31 日国家卫生计生委等 7 部门颁布的《关于建立住院医师规范化培训制度的指导意见》，人民卫生出版社推出了住院医师规范化培训规划教材第 1 版，在建立院校教育、毕业后教育、继续教育三阶段有机衔接的具有中国特色的标准化、规范化临床医学人才培养体系中起到了重要作用。在全国各住院医师规范化培训基地四年多的使用期间，人民卫生出版社对教材使用情况开展了深入调研，全面征求基地带教老师和学员的意见与建议，有针对性地进行了研究与论证，并在此基础上全面启动第二轮修订。

　　第二轮教材依然秉承以下编写原则。①坚持"三个对接"：与 5 年制的院校教育对接，与执业医师考试和住培考核对接，与专科医师培养与准入对接；②强调"三个转化"：在院校教育强调"三基"的基础上，本阶段强调把基本理论转化为临床实践、基本知识转化为临床思维、基本技能转化为临床能力；③培养"三种素质"：职业素质、人文素质、综合素质；④实现"三医目标"：即医病、医身、医心；不仅要诊治单个疾病，而且要关注患者整体，更要关爱患者心理。最终全面提升我国住院医师"六大核心能力"，即职业素养、知识技能、患者照护、沟通合作、教学科研和终身学习的能力。

　　本轮教材的修订和编写特点如下：

　　1. 本轮教材共 46 种，包含临床学科的 26 个专业，并且经评审委员会审核，新增公共课程、交叉学科以及紧缺专业教材6种:模拟医学、老年医学、临床思维、睡眠医学、叙事医学及智能医学。各专业教材围绕国家卫生健康委员会颁布的《住院医师规范化培训内容与标准(试行)》及住院医师规范化培训结业考核大纲,充分考虑各学科内亚专科的培训特点,能够符合不同地区、不同层次的培训需求。

2. 强调"规范化"和"普适性",实现培训过程与内容的统一标准和规范化。其中临床流程、思维与诊治均按照各学科临床诊疗指南、临床路径、专家共识及编写专家组一致认可的诊疗规范进行编写。在编写过程中反复征集带教老师和学员意见并不断完善,实现"从临床中来,到临床中去"。

3. 本轮教材不同于本科院校教材的传统模式,注重体现基于问题的学习(PBL)和基于案例的学习(CBL)的教学方法,符合毕业后教育特点,并为下一阶段专科医师培养打下坚实的基础。

4. 充分发挥富媒体的优势,配以数字内容,包括手术操作视频、住培实践考核模拟、病例拓展、习题等。通过随文或章节二维码形式与纸质内容紧密结合,打造优质适用的融合教材。

本轮教材是在全面实施以"5+3"为主体的临床医学人才培养体系,深化医学教育改革,培养和建设一支适应人民群众健康保障需要的临床医师队伍的背景下组织编写的,希望全国各住院医师规范化培训基地和广大师生在使用过程中提供宝贵意见。

融合教材使用说明

　　本套教材以融合教材形式出版,即融合纸书内容与数字服务的教材,读者阅读纸书的同时可以通过扫描书中二维码阅读线上数字内容。

获取数字资源的步骤

1 扫描封底红标二维码,获取图书"使用说明"。

2 揭开红标,扫描绿标激活码,注册/登录人卫账号获取数字资源。

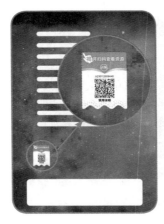
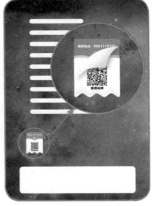

❸ 扫描书内二维码或封底绿标激活码随时查看数字资源。

❹ 下载应用或登录 zengzhi.ipmph.com 体验更多功能和服务。

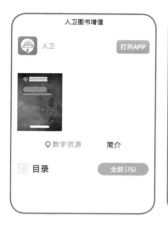

扫描下载应用

客户服务热线 400-111-8166

配 套 资 源

➢ **电子书：《住院医师英语手册》(第 2 版)** 下载"人卫 APP"，搜索本书，购买后即可在 APP 中畅享阅读。

➢ **住院医师规范化培训题库** 中国医学教育题库——住院医师规范化培训题库以本套教材为蓝本，以住院医师规范化培训结业理论考核大纲为依据，知识点覆盖全面、试题优质。平台功能强大、使用便捷，服务于住培教学及测评，可有效提高基地考核管理效率。题库网址：tk.ipmph.com。

主 编 简 介

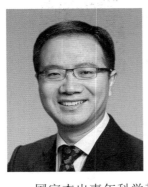

唐熠达

教授，博士生导师。现任北京大学第三医院心内科主任、血管医学研究所常务副所长、分子心血管学教育部重点实验室副主任。主要研究方向是心血管疾病介入及抗栓治疗、心血管代谢疾病的诊治等。

国家杰出青年科学基金获得者，教育部长江学者特聘教授，"新世纪百千万人才工程"国家级人选，荣获"国家卫生健康突出贡献中青年专家"称号，首都科技领军人才。

作为项目负责人先后主持多项重大国家级和省部级科研项目，包括"十二五"国家科技支撑计划、国家重点基础研究发展计划（973计划）子课题、国家自然科学基金重点项目及面上项目等。牵头多项大规模临床试验。目前共发表文章100余篇，其中在 *Circulation*，*Hepatology* 等国际著名杂志上发表SCI论文60余篇，主编、参编专著10余部。

副主编简介

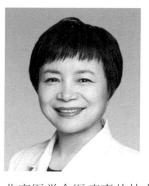

张龑

教授，硕士生导师。北京大学第三医院妇产科主任医师。主要研究方向为高危妊娠与围产感染免疫。

现任中华医学会围产医学分会感染与免疫学组委员，北京市中西医结合围产医学专业委员会委员。北京医学会医疗事故技术鉴定专业委员会鉴定专家。*Chinese Medical Journal* 与 *Fertility and Sterility* 杂志特约审稿人，北京市外国医师执业考试专家。

发表文章 30 余篇，参与国家自然科学基金项目，科技部"十三五"重大专项等研究。

副主编简介

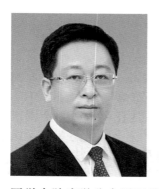

蔡世荣

教授，博士研究生导师。中山大学附属第一医院胃肠外科中心主任、胃肠外科主任，中山大学胃癌诊治研究中心副主任。

国际胃癌协会（IGCA）会员，中华医学会外科学分会胃肠外科学组委员，中华医学会肿瘤学分会胃肠肿瘤学组委员，中国抗癌协会胃癌专业委员会常委、外科学组副组长，中国抗癌协会胃肠间质瘤专业委员会委员，中国医师协会结直肠肿瘤专业委员会副主任委员。

2008年创办《消化肿瘤杂志（电子版）》，任副主编兼编辑部主任，兼任《中华实验外科杂志》《中华医学杂志》等编委。主持国家自然科学基金项目4项。

副主编简介

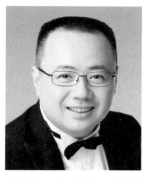

潘慧

教授，博士生导师。北京协和医院医务处处长，内分泌科主任医师。

中国医师协会医学科学普及分会副会长，中国医师协会青春期医学专业委员会常务委员，《中华行为医学和脑科学杂志》和《高校医学教学研究（电子版）》副主编，《中国医学人文杂志》和《中国卫生检验杂志》常务编委。

主持或参与国家自然科学基金面上项目，中国医学科学院医学与健康科技创新工程项目等课题 30 余项，共发表论文 300 余篇，其中 SCI 收录 70 余篇，主编参编教材专著 50 余部。获教育部高等学校科学研究优秀成果科学技术进步二等奖，高等教育国家级教学成果奖一等奖等。

副主编简介

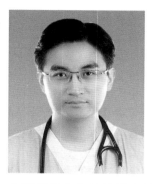

金泽宁

教授，博士生导师。现任首都医科大学附属北京天坛医院心脏及大血管中心主任。主要研究方向为各种复杂冠心病的介入治疗。

欧洲心脏病学会委员，北京医学会心血管病学分会常务委员，北京医学会心血管病学分会结构性心脏病学组副组长等。

承担国家自然科学基金项目、科技部"重大新药创制"科技重大专项等多项重大课题。荣获教育部国家科学技术进步奖一等奖。

前 言

《住院医师英语手册》第 2 版在我们的共同努力下终于与大家见面了。

本次修订在保留第 1 版"以临床实际情景为主线"的编写特色基础上,进一步优化了本书作为教科书与工具书的易用性:①收集了住院医师在第 1 版实际应用过程中提出的诸多反馈,然后将散布于各个临床场景中的重点词汇、句式、表达方式进行了系统归纳,以便于集中学习。②优选了医疗文书部分的文字材料,使其更为贴近临床应用场景。③将"英文病例报道"扩充改变为"英文论文写作"一章,适应目前住院医师学习和工作中面临的新挑战。④根据本书的文字内容,增加数字资源,构建更为立体和实用的医学英语教育素材库。

英语在医疗活动和医学科研中应用颇多,英语学术交流和医学场景下英语交流越来越常见。这就要求临床医师不仅需要在涉外诊疗工作中能够应用英语开展诊疗活动,即问诊、查体、交代病情等,还需要使用英文进行基本的学术交流,发表科研成果。住院医师经过院校的英语学习,多数已掌握基本的单词和语法,具备大学英语四、六级的水平,但由于传统的教学模式较少关注实践应用,很多年轻医师无法在临床诊疗和学术活动中熟练地使用英语。此外,医学英语作为一种专业性交流方式,特定的医学单词、术语,以及问诊和交代病情中的表述方式也是需要关注的。

2 版教材延续了上版"以医学英语为中心,以实际

13

应用为重点"的编写原则和"以临床实际情景为主线"的编写特色，并做了一些改进，以期更好地满足住院医师教学培训的需求。本教材所面向的是承担大量临床工作的住院医师，特别强调简洁性和实用性。希望本教材能够为住院医师提供专业英语训练，同时也能够成为住院医师在实际应用中的"口袋参考书"。

在本书的编写过程中得到了各位编委及同事的大力支持，参与调研的住院医师也提出了许多宝贵意见和建议，在此表示诚挚的感谢。本书打破了传统医学英语的教学模式，尝试进行全方位的创新，也难免不尽完善，请广大读者批评指正。

唐熠达

2021.11

目　录

第一章　病史采集与交代病情常用句型·················1

Chapter 1. Sentence Patterns in Medical History
　　　　　 Taking and Communication ··········1

　1．个人信息 ·······································1

　2．主诉与现病史问诊 ·····························1

　3．既往史 ···6

　4．个人史 ···7

　5．月经、婚姻和生育史 ···························7

　6．家族史 ···8

　7．系统回顾 ·······································8

　8．体格检查常用指示用语 ·························9

　9．体格检查基本步骤 ····························11

　10．各系统检查示例 ·····························12

第二章　各系统常见疾病的问诊和查体···············15

Chapter 2. History Taking and Physical
　　　　　 Examinations ························15

　1．呼吸内科 ·····································15

　2．心血管内科 ···································26

　3．消化内科 ·····································37

　4．肾脏内科 ·····································59

　5．血液内科 ·····································65

　6．内分泌科 ·····································73

　7．风湿免疫科 ···································84

　8．神经内科 ·····································92

9. 骨科 ……………………… 102

10. 胸心外科 ……………… 112

11. 神经外科 ……………… 117

12. 妇产科 ………………… 123

13. 儿科 …………………… 147

第三章　病历书写及病例报告写作 ……… 160
Chapter 3. Medical Record and Case Report
　　　　　　Writing …………………… 160

1. 病历内容 ……………… 160

2. 英文病历常用表述方式 … 161

3. 病历示例 ……………… 173

4. 其他医疗文书 ………… 194

5. 病例报告写作 ………… 242

第四章　英文论文写作 ……………… 255
Chapter 4. English Thesis Writing ……… 255

1. SCI 及影响因子简介 …… 255

2. 医学论文的格式和内容 … 257

3. 论著论文撰写原则及示例 … 262

4. 投稿及修稿程序 ……… 277

5. 投稿示例 ……………… 281

6. 医学文献阅读的策略与技巧 …… 285

附录　医学英语构词法 ………………… 289
Introduction to Medical Terminology ……… 289

第一章 病史采集与交代病情常用句型
Chapter 1. Sentence Patterns in Medical History Taking and Communication

1. 个人信息 Personal Details

How old are you?

What's your occupation?

Would you mind to tell me what you are doing for living?

Could you tell me about your marriage status, please?

2. 主诉与现病史问诊 Chief Complaint

It includes the following aspects: ①Onset and duration of the disease. ②Main symptoms, location and their character. ③Etiology and provoking factors. ④Evolution of disease. ⑤Associated symptoms. ⑥Treatment and its effects. ⑦General condition, especially the dietary habit.

病情陈述者为本人时

What's troubling you?

What seems to be your trouble?

What seems to be bothering you?

What brings you to the clinic?

What happened to your leg?

Now I want to know more details about your disease. Please sit down and answer my questions.

How did it happen? Did you hurt yourself?

Could you tell me more about how you injured your elbow?

How long have you been like this?

Were there any inducements?

Did you notice anything associated with when this trouble starts?

Did you go to see doctor and do some examinations?

Were there any pain or difficulty when moving your right arm or walking?

Did you notice any deformity, abnormality, wound or bleeding of your right elbow or buttock at the time?

Did you use other medications?

What was the dose of them?

What about the effects of these medications?

Did you change the medications?

Did you do anything to relieve the pain?

Could you sleep without pain medications yesterday?

Do you have pain in other parts of your body?

Did you experience severe pain and numbness in your right hand and fingers?

Did you suffer from the side effect of this medication?

Why did you change the regimen?

Were there some other symptoms that happened after adjusting the regimen?

What about your symptoms?

When did the chest congestion happen? How did

you relieve the chest congestion?

What about your eyesight?

Are there other symptoms that occurred recently?

What about your diet and rest?

What about your stool, urine and nocturia?

I need to ask you a few more questions and then examine you before I can tell you for sure. Can you grasp your right hand and move the elbow?

How are you going these days?

Did you do ... from the beginning to now as we have instructed you before?

Did you have any accidents last month, such as falls, knee sprains and so on?

Did you seek help from a physiotherapist?

Did you have warmth or swelling of your ...?

Have you found anything associated with when this trouble starts?

Have you taken any medications intake recently?

Did you eat many sea foods during the trip, and are you allergic to sea foods?

In any condition did you feel better or worse?

How may I help you?

Did you take your temperature?

How often do you feel feverish?

Do you have any other symptoms or problems apart from fever?

Do you feel hot and cold?

Any problems with your water work or bowels?

Have you noticed anything or any symptoms that led to the swelling? For example, cold?

What time of the day is the swelling worse?

How much water or fluid are you drinking per day?

How much urine are you passing per day?

Do you have any discomfort urinating or passing water?

Have you gained or lost any weight?

Do you have any other symptoms, like nausea, vomiting, palpitations, or short of breath?

Have you taken any medications or received any treatment since being unwell?

How long have you had this problem or these symptoms?

Is the pain there all the time?

Does anything make the pain worse? For example, on exertion.

Does the pain move to anywhere else?

Have you ever received any treatment before you came to the hospital?

When did your symptoms begin?

Is the pain there all the time or does it come and go?

Can you lie flat in bed?

Is the pain and breathing worse when you get up to walk?

Do you feel better when you lie on bed?

You should be admitted to hospital so that your treatment can start at once.

Does anything make it better or worse?

Did you bring up anything with your cough?

What color was the phlegm?

How bad is the cough?

Do the symptoms come on like an attack or develop more gradually?

Can he lie flat?

Do his lips turn(become) blue?

Is it worse any particular time of the year?

Has he ever had asthmatic attacks?

Please can you show me where on your tummy (or abdomen) you feel the pain?

Could you describe the pain, please?

How long have you had the pain?

How bad is the pain? Let's say on a 1 to 10 scale, 10 being the worst. How would you rate your pain?

Does anything bring on the pain or make it worse?

How about food, does it bring on the pain?

Have you had any similar attack before?

How is your bowel motion?

Have you lost any weight?

Do you have any other symptoms you would like to tell me about?

Have you sought medical advice since the pain started? Do they help?

Do any family members or close friends have similar symptoms?

Have you had a bowel movement today?

Do you vomit or feel nauseous?

How often do you pass stool in a day?

What does your stool look like apart from being black?

Did you do anything to relieve the pain?

Have you got fever in the recent four weeks?

Are you photosensitive?

Do you have pain on your joints or spine?

Do you have recurrent mouth ulceration?

Will your fingers or toes become white or blue when they are exposed to cold?

Is there any blood or foam in your urine?

Do you have chest pain or short of breath?

Do you have problems when sleeping?

病情陈述者非本人时

What can I do for you and your little boy?

How long ago was that?

Did you notice which part of his body hit the ground first?

Did he lose consciousness?

How long did he lose consciousness?

Was there anything else unusual about him?

Did he have any nausea or vomiting?

Did he appear alright when he regained consciousness?

Did you notice he has any twisting of his arms or legs before the accident?

Did he have any trouble in keeping balance?

Have you noticed anything different about him before the swelling?

Has he seen any doctor?

What treatment has he received?

Has he taken any medications or received any treatment since being ill?

3. 既往史 Past Medical History

Do you have any chronic diseases such as hypertension, liver disease or kidney disease?

What medicine are you taking to control your blood pressure now?

6

Have you taken any medications or received any treatment before?

Do you take any other medications on a regular basis?

May I just double check whether or not you take aspirin, warfarin, steroids or any kind of painkiller?

Did you ever have nephritis as a child?

Did you have operation?

Have you had any operations in the past?

Are you allergic to special food or drugs?

Do you have any allergies?

Do you have any other medical problems?

Do you have any other medical conditions?

4. 个人史 Social and Personal History

Do you smoke or addict to alcohol?

How much alcohol do you drink on average in a week?

How long have you been smoking?

At what age did you first begin smoking regularly?

How many cigarettes do you usually smoke a day?

Have you attempted to quit?

Have you been to the epidemic area?

Do any family members or close friends have similar symptoms?

5. 月经、婚姻和生育史 Menstrual, Marital and Childbearing Histories

Could you tell me about your marriage status, please?

When was your last menstrual period?

Do you have a regular period in recent years?

Has there been any changes in your menstruation?

How many pregnancies have you had?

Do you have abortion before?

6. 家族史 Family History

Do you or your family members have any special medical conditions, such as...?

Is there any history of diabetes in your family?

Do you have any family members or relatives who also have high blood pressure or kidney disease?

Do heart problems run in your family?

Do any illnesses run in your family?

7. 系统回顾 System Review

The purpose of this review is twofold:

①A thorough evaluation of the past and present status of each body system.

②A double check to prevent omission of significant data relative to the present illness.

- 循环系统：气短、心悸、胸痛、咳嗽、咯血、水肿、晕厥

  Circulatory System: short of breath, palpitation, chest pain, cough, hemoptysis, edema, syncope

- 呼吸系统：咳嗽、咳痰、呼吸困难、胸痛、盗汗、发热

  Respiratory System: cough, sputum, short of breath, chest pain, night sweating, fever

- 消化系统：嗳气、反酸、腹胀、腹痛、腹泻、恶心和呕吐

Alimentary System: belching, sour regurgitation, abdominal distension, abdominal pain, diarrhea, nausea and vomiting

- 泌尿系统：排尿困难、尿频和尿急、尿痛、腹痛、水肿

  Urinary System: difficulty in micturition, frequency and urgency of micturition, painful micturition, abdominal pain, edema

- 内分泌系统：心悸、怕热、多汗、烦渴、水肿、手抖、消瘦和肥胖

  Endocrine System: palpitation, heat intolerance, excessive sweating, polydipsia, edema, hand tremble, wasting and obesity

- 造血系统：乏力、头晕、心悸、出血

  Hematopoietic System: fatigue, dizziness, palpitation, bleeding

- 神经系统：头痛、晕厥、头晕和眩晕、失眠、偏瘫、失语

  Nervous System: headache, coma, dizziness and vertigo, insomnia, hemiplegia, aphasia

- 运动系统：关节痛、麻木、跛行、瘫痪

  Motor System: joint pain, numbness, claudication, paralysis

8. 体格检查常用指示用语 Common Instructions in Physical Examination

May I examine you, please?

Please take off your shirt and socks, and lie down on the bed. There is a blanket here for you to cover yourself. Let me know when you are ready, please.

Well, I will make a simple and quick check to assess the illness for you.

Let me examine quickly, unbutton your shirt and loosen your belt please.

Thank you for telling me about your problem. Next, I would like to examine your knees if you don't mind.

Please lie on your back, keep your knees bent, and try to relax.

Please lie on your back (stomach, right side, left side).

In that case, would you mind to have a pelvic examination? I think it's necessary.

Would you come toward me just a little?

Would you please lower your joint?

Let me take your temperature. Please put this thermometer under your tongue/in the axilla for ten minutes.

It is necessary to take his pulse, respiratory rate and blood pressure.

You should notice whether the patient is conscious or not.

You should notice any change of his pupils.

Look right at me, please.

Now open your mouth.

Open it just as wide as you can.

Now let me examine your nose.

Now let me take a look in your ears, first.

Just breathe easily through your mouth.

Please breathe deeply.

Take a deep breath, please.

Please say, "Ah"

Stick your tongue out.

Please sit up nice and straight.

Now put your arms on your hips.

Now over your head.

Now rest your arm on mine.

Please lift your right leg.

Does it hurt here?

Does it hurt you when I move your leg?

Does it hurt you when I touch your abdomen?

Please point to the spot where you feel the most painful.

Tell me if it hurts when I press your chest. Here?

9. 体格检查基本步骤 Procedures of Physical Examination

A detailed clinical history and physical examination are helpful in making the correct diagnosis. The history should suggest a differential diagnosis and help you to focus your physical examination. General principles of the physical examination are as follows:

(1) You should screen the bed or couch as appropriate to ensure before examining the patient.

(2) Adjust the back rest; breathless patients are more breathless lying flat.

(3) Expose the area to be examined adequately, but avoid embarrassing or chilling the patient.

(4) Make sure that the patient is warm; shivering causes muscle sounds which interfere with auscultation, and palpation with cold hands causes the abdominal muscles to contract, impairing the examination.

11

(5) Carry out your examination from the patient's right side.

(6) Gently handle any painful area.

(7) Avoid exhausting the patient from prolonged examination, especially the sick, frail or elderly. If appropriate, complete the examination in several visits.

(8) Ask the medical or nursing staff for advice about chaperoning. Young female should be chaperoned when examining.

(9) Record your examination findings systematically. Use diagrams to define the site and extent of physical findings such as swellings or the effects of trauma.

(10) Identify the patient's active problems and differential diagnoses.

10. 各系统检查示例 Examples of Examination for Each System

General: Middle-aged man walking into the ward. Speaking complete sentences. Mild diaphoretic and distressed.

Skin: No jaundice, petechiae, skin lesions or fresh rash. No palmar erythema or spider angioma.

Lymph Nodes: No enlarged superficial lymph nodes.

Heent:

Head: Hair of average texture. Scalp tender. Normocephalic/atraumatic (NC/AT).

Eyes: Conjunctiva pink, sclera anicteric.

Ears: Bilateral canal clear, TM with good cone of light.

Nose: Mucosa pink, septum midline. Bilateral frontal sinus tenderness.

Mouth: Oral mucosa pink and moist. Dentition good. Pharynx without exudates.

Neck: Neck supple. Trachea midline. Thyroid isthmus barely palpable, lobes not felt.

Breasts: Pendulous, symmetric. No masses; nipples without discharge.

Thorax and Lungs:

Inspection: No use of accessory muscle.

Palpation: Tenderness over sternum and bilateral ribs. Thorax symmetric with good excursion. Lung resonant.

Percussion: No dullness to percussion.

Auscultation: Clear to auscultation bilaterally (CTAB). No rhonchi, wheezes, rales.

Cardiovascular:

Inspection: No jugular venous distension (JVD).

Palpation: Carotid upstrokes brisk, without bruits. Apical impulse palpable in the 5th left interspace, 8cm lateral to the midsternal line. No heaving apex impulse, thrill or pericardium friction rub could be palpated.

Percussion: Cardiac dullness shown in Table 1-1.

Table 1-1　Cardiac Dullness in Normal Adult

Right/cm	Intercostal Space(ICS)	Left/cm
2～3	II	2～3
2～3	III	3.5～4.5
3～4	IV	5～6
/	V	7～9

Auscultation: Heart rate 72 beats per minute. Good S_1, S_2, no S_3 or S_4, with normal rhythm. No extra or abnormal heart sound, murmurs or pericardium friction sound. No gallops, or rubs.

Abdomen:

Inspection: Flat.

Palpation & Percussion: No tenderness or distension (NT/ND). No rebound or guarding. No hepatosplenomegaly (HSM). Murphy sign (−). No costovertebral angle tenderness (CVAT). Shifting dullness sign (−).

Auscultation: Bowel sounds active.

Genitalia & Rectal: Normal distribution of pubic hair, without externalia malformation. No scar and ulcer.

Musculoskeletal: Spine with normal curve and no tenderness. No joint deformities. Good range of motion in hands, wrists, elbows, shoulders, spine, hips, knees, ankles. Warm and without edema or clubbing. Calves supple, nontender. Pulses brisk.

Neurology: Good muscle bulk and tone. pinprick, light touch, position sense, vibration and stereognosis intact. Right rapid alternating movements (RAMs), finger-to-nose test, heel-shin test slightly stupid. Romberg (−). Gait stable. Right biceps and triceps reflex active, bilateral patellar and achilles reflex active. Abdominal reflex (+), bilateral patellar clonus(−), bilateral ankle clonus (−), bilateral palmomental reflex (−), bilateral Hoffman sign (−), bilateral Babinski sign (−), bilateral Chaddock sign (−), bilateral Oppenheim sign (−), Gordon sign (−), neck supple, Kernig sign (−), Brudzinski sign (−), Lasegue sign (−).

第二章　各系统常见疾病的问诊和查体
Chapter 2. History Taking and Physical Examinations

1. 呼 吸 内 科

体格检查中的英文对话

（1）呼吸内科常见症状/疾病：咳嗽咳痰 Cough and Expectoration

Warming up

Coughing is a defense mechanism that protects against the inhalation of noxious substances. It is a common presenting symptom in our daily clinical visits. Coughing rids the conducting airways of aspirated foreign material and excessive respiratory tract secretions. The etiology of a cough is considered in two categories: acute and chronic. 90% of chronic coughs can be explained by postnasal drip, asthma, gastroesophageal reflux, bronchiectasis, or eosinophilic bronchitis. The etiology of a patient's cough can often be deduced from the history alone. In the history, one should determine:

1) The nature of the cough. E.g., dry cough or moist cough.

2) The time and rhythm of the cough. E.g., sudden paroxysmal cough, chronic cough, with or without dyspnea, aggregation at night, in the morning, or after position change.

3) The tone of cough. E.g., hoarseness, metal tone cough, cock-like cough, silent cough.

4) The characteristics and quantity of sputum. E.g., mucous, serous, mucopurulent, purulent, hematology.

5) Any associated symptoms. E.g., fever, chest pain, sputum, hemoptysis, wheezing, clubbing, nasal congestion, heartburn.

History taking

D: Hello, how can I help you?

P: I have a cough. It's getting worse. So, I thought it would be better to come and see you.

D: *How long have you had the cough?*

P: Six months.

D: Do you have sputum?

P: No, I don't

D: Is the cough worse when you lie down?

P: No.

D: Do you have heartburn?

P: No.

D: Is the cough worse in the morning?

P: Yes, it gets worse at about 4:00 in the morning, every day.

D: *Is the cough worse when you smell something, such as the fragrance of flowers, cold air, and so on?*

P: Yes, it gets worse every time I go to the balcony, where there are a lot of flowers.

D: *Can you hear wheezing when you cough?*

P: Yes, I can.

D: *Can the cough can relieve itself?*

P: Yes, when I leave our balcony, the cough goes away slowly.

D: Have you received any treatment during the last six months?

P: I have taken antibiotics.

D: Have they worked?

P: No.

D: *Have you had any examinations before you came here?*

P: Yes, I had a bronchial dilation test.

D: What were the results?

P: Here are the reports.

D: Let me have a look. The FEV_1 was increased more than 200ml after aspiration of bronchodilator. I'd like to listen to your chest. Would you mind taking off your coat?...Breath in and out. I think we should do an in vivo allergen skin spot test and an in vitro specific IgE test, which can clarify the allergic symptoms and guide you to avoid contact with allergens and carry out specific immunotherapy as far as possible, and an X-ray to exclude other diseases and look for evidence of complications such as pulmonary infection, atelectasis, pneumothorax and mediastinal emphysema.

Communication and interpretation

D: It is likely that you have asthma and that you are allergic to pollen, which is the most common outdoor allergens causing asthma attacks. It can stimulate the airway of asthmatic patients in a hyperreactive state, which is bronchial contraction, or even spasm, causing asthma attacks.

P: Oh, that's terrible. What should I do now?

D: Asthma is a controllable disease, which is characterized by hyperresponsiveness due to the chronic allergic inflammation. It can be controlled by inhaled corticosteroids. Our aim is to achieve complete control of symptoms and protect and maintain lung function as normal as possible. First of all, I recommend that you to send all your flowers to your friends or relatives. Then begin to take the inhaled corticosteroids from now on.

P: How long do I need to inhale corticosteroids.

D: It depends on your response to the corticosteroids. If you do not have the symptoms after three months, we can reduce the dose. If you do not cough at all during the next six months and your bronchial dilation test becomes negative, we can stop the treatment. Come visit me every month. I will prescribe a first-aid medication, salbutamol, to you. You can aspirate it when you feel out of breath. Is there anything that you want to ask?

P: No, I've got it. Thank you very much. See you next month.

（2）呼吸内科常见症状 / 疾病：咯血 Hemoptysis

Warming up

Hemoptysis is defined as blood coughed out from larynx or below larynx. It is important to differentiate a pulmonary source of bleeding whether outside the lung, including the nose, nasopharynx, esophagus, or upper gastrointestinal tract. Common causes of hemoptysis include tuberculosis, bronchiectasis, pulmonary carcinoma, lung abscess, pulmonary infarction, left-sided heart failure, bronchitis, pneumonia, drugs and toxins. Hemoptysis often indicates serious underlying pathology and it always warrants a careful history and chest radiographs. Many patients also require bronchoscopy. In the history, one should determine:

1) Differentiation of hemoptysis and haematemesis.

2) Quantity and color of hemoptysis, with or without sputum.

3) Any associated symptoms. E.g., fever, chest pain, dyspnea, jaundice, or systemic hemorrhage.

4) Past medical history. E.g., pulmonary tuberculosis, bronchiectasis, arterial hypertension, smoke, and medicine taken.

History taking

D: Well, what's the trouble with you?

P: I coughed out blood.

D: When did the symptom begin?

P: This morning.

D: *Did you have nausea or vomiting before you coughed out the blood?*

P: No, I didn't have it.

D: *What was the color of the blood: bright red or dark red?*

P: Bright red.

D: *Was the blood with any sputum or food debris?*

P: Well, I coughed up some sputum before I coughed out the blood.

D: What's the nature of the sputum, I mean it's mucous, purulent or...?

P: Yellow purulent sputum.

D: *How much blood did you cough out?*

P: I coughed several times. I think that there was about 200ml!

D: Do you feel palpitation?

P: No, I didn't.

D: Do you feel cold?

P: No.

D: Did you have fever?

P: No.

D: Do you have chest pain?

P: No.

D: Do you have hematuria, melena, or a subcutaneous hemorrhage?

P: No.

D: Did you have the symptom before?

P: No, it is the first time.

D: Do you smoke?

P: No, never.

D: Do you take medication, such as warfarin or aspirin?

P: No.

D: ***Have you ever had pulmonary tuberculosis?***

P: Yes, I had it ten years ago.

D: Did you have a standard treatment for it?

P: Yes, I think so. I had antituberculotic for nine months.

D: Did you have a chest X-ray after the treatment of pulmonary tuberculosis?

P: No, I haven't had a chest X-ray for about nine years. I felt very well.

D: Please, may I examine you?

P: OK.

D: Please take off your clothes and lie on the couch.

Communication and interpretation

D: I am now going to arrange for you to have a chest

CT-scan. After that, please come back to see me.

P: Doctor, is it bad?

D: Please don't worry. The chest CT-scan shows that you had pulmonary tuberculosis before. Although you reveived nine months treatment, we can still see patchy high density shadow and strip shadow at the tuberculosis loci. The tuberculosis caused bronchiectasis in the posterior segment of the upper lobe of your left lung. The bronchiectasis was complicated with infection, which lead to your hemoptysis. The normal distribution of bronchi is dendritic, tapered from the center to the distal end. However, you can see here, distal bronchi become thicker and larger than the proximal bronchi, which means the bronchi are pathologically dilated. The CT-scan shows that the bronchiectasis is columnar, cystic, and varicose.We can see orbital signs and signia of caution in your chest CT-scan, which are the characteristics of bronchiectasis. Orbital signs show that the thickened tube wall presented parallel orbital shape. Signia of caution shows that the bronchi are thickened and larger than the bronchi accompanied by arteries, while the ratio of normal bronchi to bronchi accompanied by arteries is $0.6 \sim 0.7$.

P: Do I need to take some medicine?

D: Yes of course. Bronchiectasis may cause pleurisy, empyema, pericarditis, pulmonary heart disease, and even heart failure. Therefore, you need to accept normative treatment.

P: I totally agree with you.

D: I recommend that you be admitted to hospital to start the treatment. You need rest, sedatives, and hemostatic drugs to stop hemoptysis. As well as some antibiotics to control the infection. Maintaining smooth breathing, eliminating endocrine products in trachea, reducing sputum accumulation in airway, lungs, and bronchus, and removing places where bacteria grow and multiply, are important in infection control. Normal people expectorate by coughing, bronchial wall cartilage and mucus clearance mechanism of bronchiectasis patients has been destroyed, which means coughing can not remove sputum. X-ray examination showed that the proximal bronchi completely collapsed when coughing. Sputum can not be discharged so it is best to use a position that allows gravity to assist drainage to make the surrounding sputum flow to the larger bronchial hilum and then cough out. Nurses will give you expectorants to make sputum thinner and easier to cough up to alleviate bronchial infection and systemic toxicity and help you to expel sputum out of the body, and if necessary, with aerosol inhalation. However, it is easy to get an infection because the physical protection barrier is disturbed due to the bronchiectasis.

P: Is there anything I can do for prevention?

D: The most important is that you should not get cold after discharge. Also, avoid fatigue, emotional fluctuations, and keep your mood at ease. Your diet should be rich in nutrition, high in protein, high calorie, and high vitamin food. Pay attention to oral hygiene, gargle in the morning, before bed and after meals. Do you any questions?

P: No, thank you very much.

（3）呼吸内科重点查体

Physical examination

Physical examination is important for the initial diagnosis. In addition, it is also the only tool immediately available for assessment of the patient in emergency conditions, such as tension pneumothorax.

1) Inspection

Ask the examinee to take the seat or lay in the supine position, fully expose the front chest, and stand in front or right side of the examinee for observation. The morphology of the thorax should be observed. When observing the shape of the thorax, attention should be paid to whether there is barrel chest or flat chest, whether the rib space is full, whether the bilateral thorax is symmetrical, etc. Normal thorax is symmetrical on both sides and oval in shape. The ratio of anterior to posterior diameter to left and right diameter is 1:1.5. The respiratory frequency, respiratory rhythm, and symmetry of clinical respiratory movement were observed. Breathing of normal adult women is mainly chest breathing, while that of normal adult men and children is mainly abdominal breathing. The breathing rhythm is uniform and regular.

2) Percussion

Palpation includes **breathing movement**, **tactile tremor**, and **pleural friction.**

Enhanced vocal fremitus is caused by enhanced vocal transmission from the tracheobronchial tree to the chest wall, which can be seen in the consolidation of lung and huge cavity in lung near pleura. The mechanism of decreased speech tremor is weakened voice transmission from the tracheobronchial tree to the chest wall, it can be seen in emphysema, obstructive atelectasis, massive pleural effusion or pneumothorax, pleural hypertrophy and adhesion, and chest wall subcutaneous emphysema. Pleural friction can be seen in the cellulose exudation phase of pleurisy and uremia.

3) Percussion sounds

Resonance is the percussion sound of normal lung.

Dullness or Flatness are observed when the gas content is reduced in the lung, such as atelectasis, pneumonia, tuberculosis, or pulmonary embolism. However, diseases such as lung cancer, lung abscess, or pulmonary cyst disease, diseases of thoracic cavity, such as pleural effusion or pleural hypertrophy, and diseases of chest wall, such as edema, have normal gas content in the lung.

Hyperresonance is pathognomonic of emphysema.

Tympany is characteristic of pneumothorax or large pulmonary cavity near the chest wall.

4) Breath sounds

Normal breath sounds include tracheal breath sounds, bronchial breath sounds, bronchovesicular breath sounds, and vesicular breath sounds.

Pathological breath sounds:

Weakness or disappearance of vesicular breath sounds is auscultated when the respiratory movement, alveolar ventilation, or alveolar elasticity is reduced.

Enhancement of vesicular breath sounds is auscultated when the respiratory movement, alveolar ventilation, or alveolar elasticity is enhanced, such as after physical activity, hyperthyreosis, or severe anemia.

24

Prolonged expiration sounds are characteristics of asthma or emphysema.

Discontinued breath sounds can be heard when the gas enters unevenly into the alveoli, such as pneumonia or tuberculosis.

Rough breath sounds can be auscultated when the bronchus are not smooth, which leads to disturbance of the airflow, such as bronchitis or early stage of pneumonia.

Tubular breath sounds are characteristics of lung consolidation, larger lung cavity, or atelectasis.

Additional breath sounds:

Moist crackles could be divided into four types: coarse, medium, fine (including Velcro rales), and crepitus according to the diameter of airway and the amount of secretion. Coarse crackles are best heard in bronchiectasis or lung abscess. Medium bubble sound are best heard in bronchitis or bronchopneumonia. Fine moist crackles could be heard in bronchiolitis, pulmonary congestion, or lung infarction, while Velcro rales is characteristic of interstitial lung disease. Crepitus can be heard in bronchiolitis, alveolitis, or lung congestion.

Rhonchi is formed when the airway is narrowed in several conditions, such as airway spasm, sputum, neoplasm in the airway, or external pressure stenosis of the airway... It could be classified as sonorous and sibilant.

（4）重点语句

Cough and expectoration

How long have you had the cough?

Is the cough worse when you smell something, such as the fragrance of flowers, cold air, and so on?

Can you hear the wheezing when you cough?

Can the cough relieve itself?

Have you had any examinations before you came here?

Hemoptysis

Did you have nausea or vomiting before you coughed out the blood?

What's the color of the blood: bright red or dark red?

Was the blood with any sputum or food debris?

How much blood did you cough out?

Have you ever had pulmonary tuberculosis?

2. 心血管内科

（1）心血管内科常见症状 / 疾病：胸痛 Chest Pain

Warming up

Chest pain is one of the most common reasons for seeking care in the emergency department (ED). In a typical group of patients undergoing evaluation for chest pain in EDs, about 15% to 25% have acute myocardial infarction or unstable angina. A small percentage of patients have other life-threatening problems, for instance, pulmonary embolism or acute aortic dissection. However, most patients are diagnosed with a non-life threatening cardiac disease, such as pericarditis, or with a diagnosis of a non-cardiac-related condition, including disorders of pulmonary (e.g. pleuritis, pneumonia, spontaneous pneumothorax), disorders of the abdominal viscera (e.g. gastroesophageal reflux disease), musculoskeletal syndromes and psychological conditions. The difficulty lies in discriminating between patients with acute cooronary syndrome(ACS) or other life-threatening conditions, from those with non-cardiovascular, nonlife threatening chest pain.

History taking

D: Hello, madam, how may I help you?

P: I have chest pain sometimes, so I thought I should come see you.

D: When did the symptoms begin?

P: 3 years ago, and it bothered me again last night.

D: How often?

P: Typically, once a month, but recently it has been about twice a week for the past two months.

D: *How long does it last?*

P: Usually last for several seconds, but lately it has lasts for a few minutes, but generally no more than 30 minutes.

D: *What kind of pain is it: dull, squeezing, tightening or choking?*

P: Hmm...It's a crushing pain. It feels like there's a heavy weight on my chest.

D: *Where on your chest is the pain?*

P: Here, behind the breastbone.

P: It is difficult to describe the localization of the chest pain accurately. However, the pain usually starts in the middle of my chest and frequently spreads to both sides of the front part of my chest, but more severe on the left side.

D: ***Does it radiate to the neck, to the arm, or to the back?***

P: It usually radiates down the ulna of the left arm and produces a tingling sensation in the left wrist, hand, and fingers.

D: ***Is the pain associated with other symptoms like sweating, nausea, vomiting, or short of breath?***

P: Sometimes I felt extreme weakness, dizziness, and palpitations.

D: ***What activities cause your chest pain?***

P: It is typically caused by exercise, emotional stress, cold weather, eating a large meal, and sometimes it even happens when I lie in bed.

D: ***Does the pain ease with rest?***

P: Yes.

D: Have you taken the trinitrin nitroglycerin（or tablet under the tongue）, and if so, how quickly does it help relieve the chest pain?

P: Yes, I usually take one under the tongue, and the symptoms disappear quickly.

D: ***Have you received any tests or treatment before coming here?***

P: I did an ECG check in our local clinic last year, but the doctor said it was normal.

D: How old are you?

P: 60 years old.

D: Do you smoke?

P: No.

D: Do you have high cholesterol, high blood pressure, or diabetes?

P: No, none of them.

D: Have any of your family relatives had the above disorders or any heart disease?

P: No.

D: Would you mind taking off your coat and lie on the bed? I will give you a physical examination.

Communication and interpretation

D: It is likely that you have angina, the classic manifestation of coronary heart disease, which usually occurs in the setting of coronary atherosclerosis, coronary spasm, or other less common causes of impaired coronary blood flow. This results with the supply of myocardial oxygen being inadequate for the demand.

P: Oh, that's so terrible! What should I do now?

D: I am now going to arrange for you to have a series of clinical examinations. First you need an electrocardiography (ECG) testing, and the specific ST-segment and T wave abnormalities in ECG strongly suggest myocardial ischemia. However, normal findings on an ECG do not exclude the possibility of coronary heart disease (CHD), and it's possible you may need to do an exercise treadmill test to check for any blockages of your heart arteries. Additionally, you should undergo measurement of biomarkers of myocardial injury, including cardiac troponin T or I (cTnT or cTnI), creatine kinase MB isoenzyme (CK-MB). Finally, other examinations, such as a chest X-ray radiograph, echocardiography, multi-CT coronary angiography, or percutaneous coronary angiography would be undergoing for efficient and rapid evaluation and differential diagnosis.

P: How to treat it when I am diagnosed as CHD?

D: Routine administration of antiplatelet medications (aspirin, clopidogrel or ticagrelor), sometimes combined with anticoagulant therapy, statins, beta blockers, angiotensin converting enzyme(ACE) inhibitors or angiotensin II receptor-blockers (ARBs), and nitrates to patients with CHD was proposed to control symptoms and reduce mortality. Also, lifestyle changes are also important. Once a severe coronary arterial stenosis has been ruled out, you may need surgery, a procedure called percutaneous coronary intervention (PCI). After balloon pre-dilation, the stent would be deployed in the stenosis lesion of coronary artery. The affected coronary artery would be reperfused. It is a minimally invasive surgery and all the procedures would be conducted through a tiny tube that props open peripheral arteries. The stent is usually permanent and made of metal. The procedure usually takes less than 2 hours. You'll probably stay overnight at the hospital. Is there anything that you wish to ask?

P: No. I got it. Thank you very much.

（2）心血管内科常见症状 / 疾病：呼吸困难 Dyspnea

Warming up

Dyspnea is commonly due to cardiovascular or pulmonary diseases. The perception of dyspnea varies based on behavioral and physiologic responses. Most cases of dyspnea result from asthma, heart failure, myocardial ischemia, chronic obstructive pulmonary disease, interstitial lung disease, pneumonia, or psychogenic disorders.

The etiology of dyspnea is multi-factorial in about one-third of patients. Initial testing in patients with chronic dyspnea includes chest radiography, electrocardiography, spirometry, complete blood count, and basic metabolic panel. Computed tomography of the chest is the most appropriate imaging study for diagnosing suspected pulmonary causes of chronic dyspnea. To diagnose pulmonary arterial hypertension or certain interstitial lung diseases, right heart catheterization or bronchoscopy may be needed.

History taking

D: Hello, sit down, please. What brought you into the hospital today?

P: Recently, I have had difficulty in catching my breath.

D: How long have you been like this?

P: It started 2 years ago, but it was not severe and I could carry on as usual. However, the past 2 months I have felt short of breath, especially when I walk for long time.

D: How old are you?

P: 65.

D: *Have you ever had heart disease, tracheitis, hypertension, or diabetes mellitus?*

P: I had a myocardial infarction 10 years ago, and two stents were implanted in my heart.

D: Have you had any treatment since then?

P: Aspirin, statins, nitrates.

D: Have you received any treatment for your exertional dyspnea before?

P: No.

D: Do you smoke?

P: Yes, I've been smoking for more than 20 years with 5～10 cigarettes per day.

D: ***Do you have any problem on sleeping?***

P: My sleep is disrupted due to shortness of breath when I lay on my back, so I prefer to sleep with the head elevated.

D: How many pillows do you use for sleeping?

P: Two. I have had to start sleeping on my side at night.

D: Have you noticed any swelling of your ankles or legs?

P: Hmm...I have noticed I have started to have swelling in my ankles.

D: ***Have you noticed any other symptoms lately?***

P: It is associated with loss of appetite, fatigue, and heart palpitations.

D: Is your dyspnea getting worse, better, or staying about the same in the last 2 months?

P: I think it is getting worse. At the beginning, I could not catch my breath when I exerted myself, then I had trouble breathing when I slept as well, and now I wheeze when I'm at rest (orthopnea).

D: ***Have you had any severe coughing in the past 2 months?***

P: Sometimes in the morning, but it is not often.

D: ***Do you bring up anything when you cough?***

P: Er... most of the time I coughed up phlegm, but not a lot of it.

D: What color was the phlegm?

P: White.

D: Does heart disease run in your family?

P: Yes, my father died of a heart attack, and my sister has high blood pressure.

D: Please, may I examine you?

P: Ok.

D: Please off your clothes except your underwear, lie on the bed. I'm going to do a quick exam if that is okay with you.

Communication and interpretation

D: I am going to arrange for you to have a echocardiography, blood tests, electrocardiography, and chest radiography. These tests are to help us to find out what is causing your symptoms, so that we can advise you the best treatment to make you feel better. After that, please come back and see me for a follow-up appointment.

P: Doctor, is this part of the reports? Is it that bad?

D: There's no need to worry at this stage. Now, according to your history and examinations, you may be suffering from heart failure. That means the heart is unable to pump sufficient blood flow to meet the body's needs. It can be caused by coronary artery disease, including your previous myocardial infarction (heart attack), and the infection may have aggravated the condition.

P: Doctor, what should I do next?

D: First don't drink too much water and don't eat a salty diet. Now you may need some medications to help you relieve your symptoms of dyspnea and prevent fluid retention. You should take it on time, and you might need to see a doctor regularly for follow-up appointments. Do you have any questions?

P: No. I got it. Thank you very much.

（3）心血管内科重点查体

1) Assessing the pulse and blood pressure

Rate: Normally ranges between 60 and 90 beats per minute. Rate >100 indicates tachycardia and <60 indicates bradycardia. A pulse deficit (pulse rate < heart rate due to non-conducted heart beats) suggests atrial fibrillation.

Rhythm: Normally regular but quickens during inspiration (sinus arrhythmia). An irregular rhythm is usually due to ectopic beats or atrial fibrillation.

Blood pressure: Measure the blood pressure with the patient sitting or lying comfortably and relaxed, with the upper arm at the level of the heart. Check the blood pressure after the patient has been standing for several minutes to look for postural hypotension. This is common in patients with salt depletion, autonomic neuropathy, hypotensive drug therapy, or vasovagal syncope.

2) Heart and added sounds

The first heart sound (S_1) comprises mitral (M_1) and tricuspid (T_1) valve closure. The two components usually are best heard at the lower left sternal border in younger subjects.

The second heart sound (S_2) comprises aortic (A_2) and pulmonic (P_2) valve closure. The individual components are best heard at the second left interspace with the patient in the supine position.

The third heart sound (S_3) imparts a typical cadence to the heart sounds S_1-S_2-S_3. A third heart sound

(S_3) occurs during the rapid filling phase of ventricular diastole. An S_3 may be normally present in children, adolescents, and young adults, but indicates systolic heart failure in older adults and carries important prognostic weight. A left-sided S_3 is a low-pitched sound best heard over the LV apex with the patient in the left lateral decubitus position, whereas a right-sided S_3 is usually heard at the lower left sternal border or in the subxiphoid position with the patient supine and may become louder with inspiration.

The fourth heart sound (S_4) is coincident with atrial contraction and thus precedes S_1. It is low pitched and imparts a typical cadence to the heart sounds 'da-lup-dup'. It is often due to hypertension.

An opening snap is pathognomonic of mitral stenosis. It occurs soon after the second heart sound, is high pitched and best heard with the diaphragm between the apex and the left sternal edge.

A pericardial friction rub is characteristic of pericarditis. It is a creaking sound like walking on firm snow, best heard with the patient's breath held. It often has three components sounding like 'chi-te-chi'.

3) Examination of cardiac murmurs

Heart murmurs result from audible vibrations caused by increased turbulence and are defined by their timing within the cardiac cycle. Not all murmurs indicate valvular or structural heart disease.

Murmurs can be characterized in the following manner:

Location: the area over which a murmur is best heard depends upon the position of the heart valve or defect and the direction of blood flow.

Radiation: the direction of a murmur's rad action follows the direction of blood flow through the heart valve or cardiac defect.

Pitch: pitch may be characteristic. As a rule, the greater the pressure gradient, the higher the pitch. The murmur of mitral stenosis is low pitched and that of aortic incompetence high pitched.

Timing: murmurs are usually either systolic or diastolic; occasionally, murmurs extend through both systole and diastole, e.g. the continuous murmur of a patent ductus arteriosus.

Intensity: the loudness of a heart murmur is a relatively poor index of its clinical significance.

（4）重点语句

Chest Pain

How long does it last?

Where on your chest is the pain?

Is the pain associated with other symptoms like sweating, nausea, vomiting, or short of breath?

What kind of pain is it: dull, squeezing, tightening or choking?

Does it radiate to the neck, to the arm, or to the back?

What activities cause your chest pain? Have you received any tests or treatment before coming here?

Dyspnea

Have you ever had heart disease, tracheitis, hypertension, or diabetes mellitus? Do you have any problem on sleeping?

Have you noticed any other symptoms lately?

Have you had any severe coughing?

Do you bring up anything when you cough?

3. 消 化 内 科

（1）消化内科常见症状/疾病：腹痛 Abdominal Pain

Warm up

Abdominal pain is a frequent complaint that accounts for nearly 10 percent of all visits to the emergency department. The etiology of abdominal pain includes gastrointestinal disease (in most cases) or extra-intestinal conditions. The latter refers to disorders of the abdominal wall, thorax, genitourinary tract, or spine. In unusual circumstances some systematic diseases, such as diabetes mellitus, can also cause abdominal pain. Gastrointestinal disorders associated with abdominal pain include peptic ulcer disease, gallstone, pancreatitis, mesenteric ischemia, appendicitis, inflammatory bowel disease, infectious colitis, neoplasms, etc. Owing its numerous etiology and complicated pathogenesis, the evaluation of abdominal pain requires a thorough history, detailed physical exam, thoughtful diagnostic tests, and comprehensive clinical reasoning. Patients with acute abdominal pain should be evaluated promptly to exclude conditions warranting a surgical operation. Chronic abdominal pain that has been present for months or years is most likely functional in origin, including irritable bowel disease and centrally mediated abdominal pain.

History taking

D: Good morning. How can I help you?

P: Good morning, doctor. I am afraid I have a stomachache.

D: I am sorry to hear that. Can you show me where the pain is?

P: Here (pointing to epigastrium).

D: Please tell me more about the pain. ***What does it feel like?***

P: Oh, it's very bad, and it also hurts my back.

D: ***Is it a tearing pain?***

P: No.

D: ***Is it a cramping pain?***

P: No. I would say it is dull and sometimes burning.

D: ***How long have you had this pain?***

P: Almost two weeks. It just does not go away!

D: ***How bad is the pain? On a scale from 1 to 10, with 10 being the worst pain and 0 no pain at all. How would you rate it?***

P: I would say four or five out of 10.

D: ***Does eating worsen the pain?***

P: No. Quite the contrary, it hurts mostly during late nights and early mornings when my stomach is empty.

D: Would you say that eating alleviates the pain?

P: Yes, I think so.

D: Have you had similar symptoms before?

P: No, but my belly bloats up from time to time.

D: I see. What about your bowel movements?

P: Same as before, no change.

D: Have you lost any weight over the last two weeks?

P: I don't think so.

D: *Have you sought medical advice since the pain started?*

P: Yes. The doctor gave me Talcid and other pills to kill the pain.

D: Are they helpful?

P: A little bit, but not much.

D: *Do you take any other medications on a regular basis?*

P: No.

D: Do you take aspirin, warfarin, steroids or any other painkillers?

P: No.

D: Do you drink?

P: Well, I have a beer or two occasionally. Just social drink, you know, no big deal.

D: Good. Do you smoke?

P: One pack a day for about ten years.

D: Do you have any family members or close friends with similar symptoms?

P: No.

D: Do you have any other symptoms?

P: No, I think that is all.

D: Thank you. I think we have done the history here. May I examine you?

P: Ok, doctor.

D: Please lie on your back, keep your knees bent, and relax. Make yourself comfortable.

Communication and interpretation

P: What do you think is wrong with me, doctor?

D: I think the most probable diagnosis is peptic ulcer

disease. ***I recommend an endoscopy and ultrasound scan of your abdomen to make sure.***

P: I don't know. I mean, I am OK with ultrasound, but an endoscopy sounds scary. Is it absolutely necessary?

D: Well, certainly there are other options, but to my view, they are not as good as endoscopy. For example, ***we can give you an X-ray barium meal instead***, which requires you to drink some thick fluid allowing for evaluation of the movements of the stomach. ***However, it is bitter and it might miss minor abnormalities like a small ulcer, which an endoscopy can easily detect.*** Also, if indicated, an endoscopy allows for taking small samples for further tests. Also, before the endoscopy, we will give you sedation to make you sleep. You will be unaware of what is going on and will not remember it afterward.

P: Okay, it seems reasonable to do it. I will go for a sedated endoscopy.

D: Sensible choice. ***We will arrange for you to have the endoscopy and all the other tests tomorrow morning, so no food or water after 12 pm tonight.***

P: Endoscopy, blood test, and fasting after midnight. Is that all?

D: Yes. Do you have any other questions?

P: No, you have made it very clear. Thank you very much.

D: You're welcome. See you tomorrow.

（2）消化内科常见症状/疾病: 慢性腹泻 Chronic Diarrhea

Warm up

Diarrhea is a condition in which feces are discharged

frequently and in liquid form, sometimes containing mucus, pus, blood or undigested food.

Diarrhea is diagnosed if the following criteria are met: ①watery or loose stool; ②bowel movements more than three times a day; ③stool weight in excess of 200g/d.

It is important to recognize that diarrhea is not a disease but a symptom with numerous causes. Based on course diarrhea is classified into acute and chronic. Acute diarrhea, defined as lasting less than 4 weeks, accounts for the majority of diarrhea episodes. Most of these acute episodes are mild and self-limited. In contrast, the etiology of chronic diarrhea (longer than 4 weeks) is broad and variable. The evaluation of the patient with chronic diarrhea can be complex and the treatment challenging. Causes of chronic diarrhea range from organic diseases including chronic intestinal infections, inflammatory bowel disease, and neoplasms, etc., to functional bowel disorders such as irritable bowel syndrome. In a certain group of patients, diarrhea originates from systematic disease or iatrogenic causes.

History taking

D: Good morning. What brings you here today?

P: Good morning, doctor. I have been having some diarrhea.

D: I see. *How long have you had it?*

P: About six months.

D: *How many bowel movements have you had per day?*

P: Well, it varies. But on average I use bathroom four or five times a day.

D: Ok. ***What does your stool look like?***

P: It is watery, light brown in color.

D: ***Is there any mucus or blood in it?***

P: No. I don't have phlegm stool.

D: ***Is the stool black?***

P: No. It's light brown.

D: Does it stink?

P: No. I don't think so.

D: ***Do you feel urgent to use the bathroom before each bowel movement?***

P: Yes! I feel like I have to rush to the bathroom.

D: Does any tiny amount of feces comes out before you make it to the bathroom?

P: No, it never happened.

D: Good. ***Does the discomfort diminish after a bowel movement?***

P: Yes, doctor. You hit the nail on the head! When I get out of the toilet, I feel completely fine.

D: Does eating different food ever change your bowel movement?

P: Not really.

D: ***Does anything worsen or alleviate the bowel movement?***

P: Well, it may sound embarrassing, but my diarrhea does get worse when I am stressed or I feel anxiety.

D: ***Did you encounter anything stressful lately?***

P: My company is laying off employees. I am worried that I will be fired.

D: I'm sorry to hear that. That is a very difficult situation. Shall we get back to your symptoms? Has the diarrhea wakened you up at nights?

P: Never.

D: Have you taken your temperature?

P: Yes, It is normal.

D: Do you have any nausea or vomiting?

P: No, I don't.

D: ***Has your weight changed recently?***

P: No. And my appetite is good as usual.

D: That is good. Have you traveled recently?

P: About 2 weeks ago, I paid my parents a visit in another city. But I have already had diarrhea before traveling, so it's unlikely to be the cause of my diarrhea.

D: I agree. Is there any family member or close friend with similar symptoms?

P: I don't think so.

D: Do you have any other medical conditions?

P: No.

D: Are you on any regular medication?

P: No.

D: OK. I need you to untie your clothes so I can examine your stomach. Is that OK?

P: Of course. Let's do it.

D: Thank you. Please lie down in a supine position with the head resting on one pillow and arms by two sides to relax the abdominal musculature. Make yourself comfortable.

P: OK.

D: I need to expose your abdomen.

P: OK.

D: Respiration movement, visible pulsations, peristalsis, and distended veins are all normal. Show me on your stomach where it hurts the most.

P (point the painful place): Here.

D (begin gentle palpation at a site remote from the area of pain, assess muscle tone in each area and look at the patient's expressions, checking for any signs of discomfort): Is it painful here?

P: No.

Communication and interpretation

P: Doctor, what do you think is causing my diarrhea?

D: Well, several disorders can cause chronic diarrhea similar to what you have described. However, I think it is most likely due to functional bowel disorders.

P: What are functional bowel disorders? I have never heard that before.

D: It is a intestinal function disorder characterized by persistent or intermittent seizures, lack of gastrointestinal structure, and biochemical abnormalities. The onset of the disease is slow and intermittent. The occurrence or aggravation of symptoms is often related to mental factors or stress state. It is aggravated during the day and alleviates after sleeping at night. It has little effect on health, but the course of disease is long, which affects the quality of work and life of patients in varying degrees. So, don't be too nervous about it.

P: OK. What needs to be done?

D: First of all, we need to make sure that there is no structural change of your organs. So, I suggest that we run some blood tests, a stool exam, to make sure whether or not you have bloody stools, an ultrasound, and maybe a colonoscopy, which involves looking at your colon through a thin tube that contains a camera. If all those tests come back negative, then we will be certain that it is functional. Because the diagnosis of functional bowel disease is based on symptoms and excluding organic diseases. When we ensure the diagnosis, I will give you some medications for it. How does that sound?

P: I think I am ok with your plan, Doctor. Thanks. I forgot to tell you that my father had pancreatic cancer. Could I have it too?

D: Oh, I am sorry to hear that. But a pancreatic cancer is very unlikely in your case, as your symptoms do not fit it at all. Besides, some blood and imaging tests should help us exclude pancreatic cancer. So please do not worry about it.

P: Thank you very much, doctor. It is very reassuring.

D: I will give you antidiarrheal agents which can improve diarrhea. But you need to pay attention to adverse reactions such as constipation and abdominal distension. I do think your symptoms are relevant to your social stress. So try to stay optimistic, in a stable mood, and relaxed. You could try listening to music or exercising. . This will help prevent vegetative nerve dysfunction, which would result in slow gastrointestinal peristalsis, reduced secretion of digestive juice, dyspepsia and other symptoms.

P: I will take your advice, thank you so much.

（3）消化内科常见症状/疾病：消化道出血 Gastrointestinal Bleeding

Warming up

Gastrointestinal hemorrhage is a common clinical problem with a variety of causes, including bleeding from a peptic ulcer, portal hypertension, neoplasms, inflammation, and angiodysplasia, etc. The ligament of Treitz has traditionally been defined as the boundary between upper and lower gastrointestinal hemorrhage. Capsule endoscopy and small-bowel endoscopy however have revolutionized the management algorithm of small bowel bleeding, and it is clear that bleeding from the small bowel represents a distinct entity. Therefore, it seems reasonable to divide gastrointestinal bleeding into three categories: upper (proximal to the ligament of Treitz), middle (jejunum and ileum), and lower (colon and rectum) bleeding.

Gastrointestinal hemorrhage can be acute or chronic, occult (≤200ml/day) or frank. According to the amount of bleeding, gastrointestinal hemorrhage is classified into mild, moderate, severe and life-threatening. A detailed history and thorough physical examination are pivotal in the diagnosis, assessment, and management of gastrointestinal hemorrhage. The management depends on the etiology and severity of the bleeding.

History taking

Case I

D: Have a seat, please. Tell me what is troubling you.

P: Thanks doctor. I have been so weak during the past three months. And my stool has turned black in the last two days.

D: Did you vomit or feel nauseous?

P: No. I didn't vomit or have nausea.

D: *What does your stool look like?*

P: It is black and loose.

D: ***Do you have any abdominal pain?***

P: Yes. On the upper side of my belly.

D: What does the pain feel like?

P: It feels like some sort of burning and dull ache, especially after meals.

D: Does the pain go anywhere else?

P: No.

D: How long have you had this pain?

P: Well, it was on and off for about two or three years, but not always. It's never been this bad before.

D: Do you feel pain at night?

P: Yes, it happens very early in the morning.

D: ***How is your appetite?***

P: Not very good. I feel bloated most of the time.

D: ***Have you lost weight recently?***

P: Yes, about 5 kg or even more.

D: Do you have a fever or night sweats?

P: No, I don't think so.

D: Do you have any other medical conditions that we have not talked about, including liver or heart disease?

P: No.

D: Have you ever seen a doctor about the problem before?

P: No. I am just taking a pill called Talcid from a friend of mine. It used to be effective to kill the pain, but not this time.

D: What other medications are you taking?

P: Nothing regularly.

D: ***How much alcohol do you drink on average in a week?***

P: I don't drink a lot, maybe one or two glasses of

wine a week, but I smoke a lot.

D: What do you do to make a living?

P: I am a taxi driver.

D: ***Do you or your family members have any special medical conditions, such as*** cancer, hepatitis, tuberculosis or other infectious diseases?

P: No, I don't think so.

D: May I give you a physical exam?

P: Sure, doctor.

D: OK. Please take off your clothes except for underwear and lie on the examination table. You may use this blanket to cover yourself. Please let me know when you are ready.

Doctor closes the curtain for privacy...

P: I am ready, doctor.

D: OK.

Communication and interpretation

P: Doctor, is it serious?

D: Your heart rate and blood pressure are fine. However, we need to do some tests, including a blood cell counting to determine whether you have anemia, and a gastroscopy to figure out whether these is some type of structural change. It might take a couple of days. Do you have any family members with you?

P: My wife is here.

D: Good. I'll show you how to arrange the tests. I will also prescribe some medications for you.

P: Sounds good. Thank you.

A couple of days later...

P: Good morning, doctor. I feel better these days, but not completely back to normal yet. My stool is no longer black. Here are the results of my tests you asked me to do. I had my gastroscopy earlier this morning.

D: Good. Let me take a look... There is an ulcer in the stomach. You also have anemia, by this I mean you have lost some blood.

P: Do I need more tests or treatment?

D: A small piece of tissue was taken during the gastroscopy, to allow for detailed examination. The result should be back in one week.

P: Is it serious? Could it be cancer, doctor?

D: To tell the truth, I don't think so. And we have biopsied the ulcer and the report will come back next week. We will know more then. But I do recommend you repeat the gastroscopy three months later, after we finish the treatment.

P: OK, I see. Thank you, doctor.

Case Ⅱ

D: How can I help you?

P: I feel really tired the last several days. I look pale and feel exhausted. My stool looks black and is loose.

D: How long have you felt weak?

P: About two days.

D: Do you feel pain anywhere?

P: I always feel pain in my stomach (pointing to the upper abdomen), especially when I am hungry.

D: *Does anything make it better?*

P: I used to eat something to relieve the pain. I have this symptom for several years, especially in the cold weather.

D: *Have you ever seen a doctor about this before?*

P: No, I haven't. But I got some medicine from a

pharmacist.

D: ***What medications are you taking?***

P: I can't remember but it normally helps. This time it has not been working.

D: Do any of your relatives have similar problems?

P: I don't think so.

D: Do you have any liver disease?

P: No.

D: Are you vomiting at all?

P: No. I haven't been vomiting.

D: Please may I examine you?

P: OK, doctor.

D: ***Could you take off your clothes except for your underwear and lie on the couch.*** You may use this blanket to cover yourself. Please let me know when you are ready.

P: OK.

P: I am ready, doctor.

D: OK.

Communication and interpretation

D: I think you are bleeding from your stomach or duodenum since your stool has turned black. It is closely related to abnormal gastric acid secretion, H. pylori infection, non-steroidal anti-inflammatory drugs (NSAID), irregular life and diet, work and external pressure, smoking, drinking and psycho-psychological factors. As a result, ***you are losing blood, which makes you look pale with low blood pressure and high heart rate.*** I recommend you be admitted to hospital for urgent treatment and further tests.

P: Will I need to stay in the hospital for a long time?

D: Usually a few days but it may be longer depending on how you are and what we find out from the tests. If you agree to be admitted to the hospital, please make an in-patient registration over there.

After one day (on the ward)

D: Do you feel better today?

P: Yes, of course. After the transfusion, I feel much better.

D: Your hemoglobin was only 6g/dl, almost half the normal amount due to the bleeding.

P: You are right, doctor. I had a gastroscopy yesterday. The endoscopist told me that I was bleeding from a big ulcer in the duodenum. Luckily the bleeding had already stopped before the gastroscopy. Thank you very much for helping me.

D: You are welcome. Common complications of duodenal ulcer are perforation, bleeding, and obstruction due to repeated ulcer and duodenal stenosis. Therefore, you need take some medicine to treat your ulcer and prevent these complications.

P: Of course, please.

D: Our goal is to control symptoms, promote ulcer healing, prevent recurrence and avoid complications. I will give you omeprazole, which is proton pump inhibitor, it can promote ulcer healing faster and has a higher healing rate. It is the first choice for the treatment of duodenal ulcer. And the combination of mucosal protective agents which can improve the quality of ulcer healing and reduce the recurrence of ulcer.

P: I have heard that a Helicobacter infection can cause the condition I have. Do I have the infection?

D: Yes, the test was positive. I will give you a course of antibiotics to eradicate the Helicobacter as well.

P: Thank you very much, doctor!

D: ***Have you passed any stool today?***

P: Not yet. I haven't eaten anything since the admission.

D: You may start to eat and drink now. Also, it is important for ulcer healing and recurrence prevention to give up bad habits, reduce the stimulation of smoking, alcohol, spicy, strong tea, coffee and some drugs. You may need to change your lifestyle.

P: I will take your advice, thank you so much.

（4）消化内科重点查体

1) Signs of chronic liver disease: Finger clubbing, gynaecomastia, leukonychia, testicular atrophy, palmar erythema, loss of axillary hair, Dupuytren's contracture, parotid enlargement, spider naevi, peripheral edema.

2) Examination of the peripheral signs of gastrointestinal disease(table2-1～table2-2)

Table 2-1　West Haven grading of hepatic encephalopathy

Stage	Alteration of consciousness
Stage 0	No change in personality or behavior's no asterixis
Stage 1	Impaired concentration and attention span sleep disturbance, slurred speech, asterixis, agitation or depression
Stage 2	Lethargy, drowsiness, apathy or aggression. Disorientation. Inappropriate behavior. Slurred speech

continue

Stage	Alteration of consciousness
Stage 3	Confusion and disorientation. Bizarre behavior Drowsiness or stupor. Asterixis is usually absent
Stage 4	Comatose with no response to voice commands Minimal or absent response to painful stimuli

Table2-2　Child-Pugh classification of prognosis in cirrhosis

Score	1	2	3
Bilirubin (pmol/L)	<34	34～50	50
Albumin (g/L)	35	28～35	<28
Ascites	None	Mild	Marked
Encephalopathy	None	Mild	Marked
Prothrombin Time (seconds)	<4	4～6	>6

Child A = Score < 7　l year survival 82%

Child B = Score 7～9　l year survival 62%

Child C = Score > 9　l year survival 42%

3) Inspection and palpation of the abdomen

①In a warm environment, ask the patient to lie down in a supine position with their head resting on one pillow and arms by two sides to relax the abdominal musculature. Make sure that the patient is comfortable.

②Expose the abdomen from xiphisternum to symphysis pubis.

③Observe any movement with respiration, visible pulsations, peristalsis, masses, striae, and distended veins.

④Inquire about any pain or discomfort before palpating the abdomen, then begin gentle palpation at a site remote from the area of pain.

⑤Assess muscle tone in each area and look at the patient's expressions, checking for any signs of discomfort.

⑥Palpate more deeply, pressing firmly in each region and characterize any mass found.

⑦Examine guarding, rebound tenderness, rigidity spasm and visible peristalsis.

4) Palpation of the abdominal organs

①Palpate the liver, trace the surface and edge of a palpable liver across the abdomen. Note its shape, size, texture and any tenderness.

②Look for tenderness overlying an inflamed gall bladder. Press the thumb under the costal margin in the midclavicular line and ask the patient to breathe in deeply. Note any sudden arrest of inspiration because of localized pain. (Murphy's sign)

③Palpate the kidneys: use a bimanual technique with one hand behind the flank and the other just beneath the costal margin in the midclavicular line. Ask the patient to breathe in deeply as the two hands gently close on the kidney. At maximal inspiration, try to flip the kidney up from below, between the two hands.

The normal spleen lies deep within ribs 9~11 and never extends beyond the midaxillary line. The splenic enlargement causes dullness to percussion over the spleen, extending into the lower chest; it is best distinguished from an enlarged kidney by percussion, movement on respiration and the inability to palpate between it and the costal margin.

5) Percussion and auscultation of the abdomen

①Percuss the abdomen to detect the presence of any ascites, mass or organomegaly.

②Percuss the upper and lower borders of the liver and spleen and around the bladder.

③Look for shifting dullness if there is any abdominal distension.

④Percuss from the midline to the flanks until the percussion turns from tympanitic to dull.

⑤Mark the boundary between the area of resonance and dullness; roll the patient towards you and wait 10 seconds for the fluid to redistribute.

⑥Percuss again: if the percussion notes in the flank changes from resonant to dull, confirm the finding by percussing back towards the midline, which should still be resonant. Listen for bowels sounds for at least 1 minute.

⑦Listen over the aorta and renal arteries for bruits.

⑧Try to elicit a succussion splash if gastric outlet obstruction is suspected. Place one hand under the ribcage in each flank and shake the patient vigorously from side to side.

Ascites is suggested by central resonance but dullness in the flanks and pelvis (shifting dullness). In contrast, pelvic masses cause displacement of the bowel to the flanks, resulting in central dullness and flank resonance.

Abdominal distension may be apparent to the patient yet undetectable by the observer (functional bloating). Visible distension may be caused by fat, flatus, feces, fetus, fluid and functional bloating. Exclude the possibilities of increased abdominal wall fat by assessing the thickness of the subcutaneous tissues on gently pinching, or by observing the shape of the abdomen as the patient sits forward.

6) Digital examination of the rectum

①Obtain the patients informed consent: offer a chaperone.

②Reassure the patient: rectal examination may be uncomfortable, but it should not be painful.

③ Place the patient in the left lateral position: ask the patient to place the buttocks at the edge of the couch with the knees drawn up.

④Use lidocaine (lignocaine) gel in the anal canal if an anal fissure is suspected.

⑤Use gloves: examine the perianal skin in a good light, looking for evidence of skin lesions, external hemorrhoids or fistulas.

⑥Lubricate the examining forefinger.

⑦Place the tip of the forefinger on the anal margin and with steady pressure on the sphincter, pass the finger gently through the anal canal into the rectum.

⑧Ask the patient to squeeze the examining forefinger with the anal sphincter, note the strength and symmetry of sphincter contraction.

⑨Palpate around the entire circumference of the rectum, note any abnormality and assess any mass systematically.

⑩Repeat the rectal examination after the patient has defecated, if in doubt about palpable masses.

⑪Examine the finger after withdrawal for the presence of blood and mucus; test the stool sample for blood using a "Hemoccult" kit.

The rectum is normally empty, with smooth, soft walls. The coccyx and sacrum can be felt through the posterior rectal wall. In the female, the cervix uteri can be felt as a firm, round mass anteriorly. Vaginal tampons or a pessary may also be felt, confusing the novice. In the male, the prostate is felt anteriorly.

The normal prostate gland is smooth with a firm consistency, and its contours are like miniature buttocks represented by a shallow median groove between the lateral lobes. Pain and tenderness over the prostate indicate prostatitis. Symmetrical enlargement suggests benign hypertrophy; asymmetrical enlargement suggests carcinoma of the prostate.

（5）重点语句

Abdominal Pain

What does it feel like?

Is it a cramping pain?

Is it a tearing pain?

How long have you had this pain?

How bad is the pain? On a scale from 1 to 10, with 10 being the worst pain and 0 no pain at all. How would you rate it?

Does eating worsen the pain?

Have you sought medical advice since the pain started?

Do you take any other medications on a regular basis?

I recommend an endoscopy and ultrasound scan of your abdomen to make sure.

We can give you an X-ray barium meal instead.

However, it is bitter and it might miss minor abnormalities like a small ulcer, which endoscopy can easily detect.

We will arrange you to have the endoscopy and all the other tests tomorrow morning, so no food or water after 12 pm tonight.

Chronic Diarrhea

How long have you had it?

How many bowel movements have you had per day?

What does your stool look like?

Is there any mucus or blood in it?

Is the stool black?

Do you feel urgent to use the bathroom before each bowel movement?

Does the discomfort diminish after a bowel movement?

Does anything worsen or alleviate after the bowel movement?

Did you encounter anything stressful lately?

Has your weight changed recently?

Gastrointestinal Bleeding

Case Ⅰ

What does your stool look like?

Do you have any abdominal pain?

How is your appetite?

Have you lost weight recently?

How much alcohol do you drink on average in a week?

Do you or your family members have any special medical conditions, such as...?

Case Ⅱ

Does anything make it better?

Have you ever seen a doctor about this before?

What medications are you taking?

Have you passed any stool today?

Please could you take off your clothes except for your underwear and lie on the couch?

You are losing blood, which makes you look pale with low blood pressure and high heart rate.

I will give you a course of antibiotics to eradicate the Helicobacter as well.

4. 肾 脏 内 科

（1）肾脏内科常见症状/疾病：水肿 Edema

Warming up

Edema is an important and common presenting symptom in daily clinical visits. Many patients worry that their edema is due to a serious kidney problem, such as renal failure. However, there is a wide variety of causes for edema, of which many are non-nephrotic origins. Nephrotic causes of edema include nephritic syndrome and renal failure. A careful history of the symptom of edema helps to determine or narrow down the causes of the patient's edema. By taking a history one should determine:

1) Age, sex, and stage of disease.

2) The characteristics of edema, whether there are predisposing factors or precursor symptoms. Information regarding initial location, chronological order and extent of edema should be obtained. Whether the rate of edema development is concave or not, whether there is pleural

effusion or ascites.

3) Accompanying symptoms

Local: skin color, temperature, tenderness, rash.

Systemic: palpitation, shortness of breath, cough, sputum, other manifestations of cardiopulmonary diseases, urine volume and color alteration, hypertension, urine examination, renal dysfunction, gastrointestinal symptoms, skin yellowing, bleeding tendency, anorexia, cold fear, slow responsiveness, constipation, etc.

4) In general, pay special attention to the change of body weight.

5) Frequency of the pain, if any. E.g., a few times a day, once a week, present all the time.

History taking

D: Hello, how may I help you?

P: I have edema, so I thought it was a good idea to come and see you.

D: When did the symptoms begin?

P: Three months ago.

D: Do you still have the edema now?

P: Yes.

D: *Does the edema begin from the eyelids or from the lower limbs?*

P: It's from my eyelid.

D: *Does the edema last all day long*?

P: It's serious in the morning and lightened in the evening.

D: *Does the edema spread to anywhere else?*

P: Yes, it spread to my legs.

D: Do you feel it in both legs equally?

P: Yes.

D: *Is there any foam in your urine?*

P: Yes, I have had foam in my urine for about 6 months.

D: *Is there color change in your urine?*

P: No.

D: *Is there any dysuria, frequent urination, or urination pain?*

P: No.

D: *Are there any rashes on your skin?*

P: No.

D: *Is there any joint pain?*

P: No.

D: *Have you received any treatment before coming here?*

P: I had a urine test.

D: What did it show?

P: Here is the report.

D: Let me have a look. There is blood and protein in your urine. I'd like to check your legs. I think we should do a blood test and repeat the urine test as well.

Communication and interpretation

D: It is likely that you have nephritis syndrome, which means injury in the kidney cells.

P: Oh, that sounds terrible! What should I do?

D: Nephritis syndrome is a group of different diseases, including the primary glomerulonephritis and secondary glomerulonephritis. But it often responds well to timely medical treatment. I recommend that you be admitted to the hospital so that we can start to treat you as soon as possible. You will have a renal biopsy. Then we will give you pills to reduce proteinuria. Depending on the biopsy results, you may also need to take immune suppressors to help control the inflammation in your kidneys. Is there anything that you would like to ask about?

P: No. I got it. Thank you very much.

（2）肾脏内科重点查体

1）Assessing the blood pressure

Blood pressure: Measure the blood pressure with the patient sitting or lying comfortably and relaxed, with the right upper arm at the level of the heart. Check the blood pressure after the patient has been standing for several minutes to look for postural hypotension. This is common in patients with salt depletion, autonomic neuropathy, hypotension drug therapy, or vasovagal syncope.

2）Renal palpation

Kidney examination is usually performed by palpation with both hands. This can be done with the patient in the supine position or the standing position.

When palpating the right kidney in the supine position, ask the patient to bend his legs. The doctor should stand on the right side of the patient and ask the patient to take a deep abdominal breath. The doctor uses his left palm to hold the patient's right waist and puts his right palm on the right upper abdomen, with the finger direction roughly parallel to the right rib edge for deep palpation of the right kidney. The patient touches the kidney with both hands when he inhales. If you touch a smooth, blunt, and round organ, it may be the lower pole of the kidney. If you can hold a larger part between your hands, you can perceive its broad bean shape slightly. At this time, patients often have soreness or nausea-like discomfort.

When palpating the left kidney, the left hand crosses the front of the patient's abdomen and lifts the left side of the waist from behind. The right palm is placed across the patient's left upper abdomen. The left kidney is palpated with both hands according to the anterior method. If the patient's abdominal wall is thicker or the movement is not coordinated so that the right hand is difficult to press to the back abdominal wall, the following method can be tried: When the patient breathes in, he impacts the back of his waist forward with his left hand. If the kidney moves down between his two hands, the right hand has the feeling cloud pushed against it, and the right hand can also use the right finger to do the impact action in the left-hand direction. The left hand can also have the same feeling and touch the kidney. If the kidney is not touched in the recumbent position, the patient can stand beside the bed. The doctor can touch the kidney with both hands before and after the patient's side.

When inflammation or other diseases occur in the kidney and urinary tract, tenderness may appear at the corresponding sites. The rib ridge and rib waist are often tender sites due to inflammatory diseases of the kidneys, such as pyelonephritis, renal abscess, and renal tuberculosis.

3）The examination method of edema

The examination method of edema is also palpation. Although visualization can detect overt edema, it is not easy to find mild edema. Pitting edema may occur after local compression, while muco edema has no tissue depression after compression, although the tissue swelling is obvious. According to the severity of edema, it can be divided into three grades: mild, moderate, and severe.

Mild: only seen in the eye, face, suborbital soft tissue, anterior tibia, or ankle subcutaneous tissue. After finger compression, a slight impression can be seen on the tissue before returning to normal.

Moderate: There are marked edema in all the tissues of the body. After finger compression, obvious or deep tissue subsidence appeared and the recovery is slow.

Severe: Severe edema of the whole body, tension and brightness of the lower body skin, and even fluid exudation.

（3）重点语句

Edema

Does the edema begin from the eyelids or the lower limbs?

Does the edema last all day?

Does the edema spread anywhere else?

Is there any foam in your urine?

Is there color change in your urine?

Is there any frequent micturition or urination pain?

Are there any rashes on your skin?

Is there any joint pain?

Have you received any treatment before coming here?

5. 血 液 内 科

（1）血液内科常见症状/疾病: 白血病 Leukemia

Warming up

Leukemia is a clonal hematological malignancy, characterized by the abnormal increase of white blood cells with variable numbers of blasts in the peripheral blood (PB) and hypercellularity with increased blasts in the bone marrow (BM) in patients. It can be divided into several subtypes. Some forms of leukemia mainly occur in children. The major subtypes of leukemia are:

1) Acute lymphocytic leukemia (ALL) is the most common type of leukemia in young children. ALL types can also occur in adults.

2) Acute myelogenous leukemia (AML) is a common type of leukemia with high prevalence in adults. It also occurs in children.

3) Chronic lymphocytic leukemia (CLL) is the most common chronic adult leukemia. The patients may feel healthy for years without any need of treatment.

4) Chronic myelogenous leukemia (CML) mainly affects adults. CML patients may have few or no symptoms for months or years before entering a phase in which the leukemia cells grow more quickly.

5) Other types. Other rarer types of leukemia exist, including hairy cell leukemia, myelodysplastic syndromes, and myeloproliferative disorders.

In our bodies, white blood cells fight against infection. They normally grow and divide in an orderly way based on the body need. Healthy blood cells after the programmed death are replaced by new cells, which are produced in the bone marrow. However, this may change when the DNA of immature blood cells, mainly white blood cells, becomes mutated in some way. This causes the blood cells to grow and divide in a redundant manner. The abnormal blood cells accumulate in blood and in surrounding tissue. These abnormal cells stop the healthy white blood cells and other cells from growing and functioning normally, by crowding out space in the blood.

History taking

D: Hello, how can I help you?

P: I found some blood spots under my skin and sometimes my nose bleeds. So, I thought I should have an examination.

D: *Can I have a look on the blood spots?*

P: Yes.

D: *Is there any other place where you notice irregular bleeding?*

P: Yeah, I observe bleeding from my gums while brushing the teeth. I also have frequent nose bleedings.

D: When did it start?

P: One month ago.

D: Have you had anything like this before?

P: No.

D: *Do you have fever?*

P: Yes.

D: Do you have a cough?

P: Yes.

D: *Do you feel bone or joint pain?*

P: Yes, sometimes I have sternum tenderness.

D: *Do you feel tired?*

P: Yes, I am always feeling exhausted.

D: Do you feel nausea?

P: Yes. I have lost my appetite and I found that I lost a lot of weight.

D: *Did someone from your family suffer from similar condition?*

P: No.

D: *Did you take any medication recently?*

P: No.

D: Do you have other health problems, such as liver or kidney disease?

P: No.

D: Have you been examined before coming here?

P: Yes, I had the blood routine test.

D: What were the results?

P: Here are the reports.

D: Let me have a look. You have the anemia. Your blood platelet is very low and the level of white blood cells is high. I think we should do a bone marrow cytology test, cytochemical examination and immunological examination to help assess your condition.

After examination is done

D: Based on my assessment and results from the bone marrow cytology test, cytochemical examination, and immunological examination, I think you need to stay in hospital for further monitoring and treatment.

Communication and interpretation

P: Hi doctor, could you tell me more about my condition?

D: I am so sorry to tell you that it is likely that you have leukemia.

P: Oh, that's terrible! What exactly is leukemia?

D: Leukemia is a type of cancer affecting the blood cells. There are three sorts of blood cells in the body, red blood cells (which carry oxygen), white blood cells (which are responsible for fighting infection), and platelets (which help control bleeding). In bone marrow, immature cells multiply and mature into red cells, white cells, and platelets. As they mature, they are released into the bloodstream. In leukemia, the white blood cells, instead of growing and developing normally, grow out of control and do not mature. Cancer cells accumulate in bone marrow and other hematopoietic tissues. Cancer cells also infiltrate to non-hematopoietic organs, while inhibiting normal hematopoietic function.

Because your platelets are low to stop the bleeding and your body is susceptible to infection due to less white blood cells, I recommend that you stay in the hospital so that your treatment can be started as soon as possible. These conditions are very dangerous.

P: What's the cause of the bleeding?

D: Due to the uncontrolled growth of immature white blood cells. They can crowd the bone marrow preventing it from producing healthy platelets. When your platelets decrease, your blood clotting ability is weakened.

P: I've never been sick before. At what age do people get these?

D: Leukemia typically occurs in adults older than 55, but it is also the most common cancer in children younger than 15.

P: Will my children suffer from the same disease as me?

D: It is hard to say, but clinical data revealed that leukemia demonstrates familial aggregation.

P: How about the treatment?

D: We will use chemotherapy, consisting of traditionally "cytotoxic" drugs, to destroy rapidly dividing cells including cancer cells. If possible, we'll perform hematopoietic stem cell transplantation. Do you have more questions?

P: No, I got it. I'll take your advice. Thank you very much.

（2）血液内科常见症状 / 疾病：贫血 Anemia

Anemia is a condition in which the number of red blood cells (RBCs) or the amount of hemoglobin in the blood is below 'normal' for age and sex of the individual. It is thus defined as a decrease in the red cell mass and is usually discovered and quantified by measurement of the RBC count, hemoglobin (Hb) concentration, and hematocrit (Hct). Anemia is considered in males when Hb levels are lower than 12 g/dl and in females with Hb levels less than 11 g/dl. The main reasons of anemia are: ①decreased production of red blood cells, ②loss of blood (hemorrhage) or ③break-down of red blood cells (hemolysis). Anemia is a symptom of disease that requires an investigation to determine the underlying cause.

The symptoms of anemia depend on its severity, its rate of occurrence and presence of co-existing diseases. If it occurs gradually (chronic anemia) as in nutritional deficiency or chronic disease, the body is able to adapt itself and the person may be able to function even with a low hemoglobin level. On the other hand, if anemia occurs in a short period of time (acute anemia) due to bleeding or red cell breakdown, the symptoms appear rapidly. Anemia is accompanied by symptoms such as feeling of tiredness, lack of stamina, light-headedness and shortness of breath. When anemia results from breaking down of the red blood cells, there may also be jaundice, which results in pale color of the skin and eyes.

History taking

D: Hello, sit down please. What's wrong?

P: I took a medical examination recently and it said I am anemic.

D: OK. How old are you?

P: 35 years old.

D: ***Do you feel more tired than usual?***

P: Yes. Sometimes after a small household chore, I feel tired and need to take a rest. I also feel breathless when I go upstairs.

D: Do you have chest pain?

P: No, I don't experience any chest pain.

D: Do you have a cough?

P: No.

D: Do you have a family history of anemia?

P: No.

D: ***Have you noticed any change in your stool color or blood in your stool?***

P: I never noticed them, but I think it is normal.

D: Are you having regular menstruation?

P: No, they lasted for almost ten days in recent months.

D: Are they heavy?

P: Umm, a little.

D: Do you eat meat?

P: I rarely eat meat to stay slim.

D: Have you had some medication or vitamins recently?

P: No, I haven't.

D: ***Did you have any health problems before?***

P: No.

D: Can I see your examination report?

P: Of course. Here you are.

D: After my assessment and reviewing the results from the blood routine test, I think you need to take some drugs and adjust your eating habits.

Communication and interpretation

P: Doctor, is it serious?

D: Don't worry. Anemia is the most common blood condition. Based on hemoglobin level it is classified as mild (up to 10 g/dl), moderate (5~10 g/dl), and severe (less than 5g/dl). Based on your examination results, I think you are suffering from mild anemia.

P: What's the cause of anemia, doctor?

D: From the report, I assume that iron deficiency caused your anemia. This is the most common type of anemia worldwide. Iron deficiency anemia is caused by a shortage of iron in your body. Your bone marrow needs iron to make hemoglobin. Without adequate iron, your body can't produce enough hemoglobin for red blood cells. You lose lots of blood during periods and you haven't eaten meat. Both of them lead to the deficiency of iron in your body.

P: What is the treatment?

D: Don't worry. I'll give you iron tablets. And you need to revisit the clinic after 12 weeks for a blood routine test.

P: What should I do next to prevent this from happening again?

D: An iron-rich diet can help you alleviating the symptoms and prevent you from iron deficiency anemia. The following foods are high in iron: iron-fortified cereals and breads, dark-green leafy vegetables (such as curly kale and watercress), pulses and beans, brown rice, white and red meats, nuts and seeds, fish, tofu, eggs, and dried fruits such as apricots, raisins, and prunes. You should also eat some meat to keep a balanced nutrition.

P: OK. Thank you, doctor.

（3）血液内科重点查体

A physical examination is suggested to focus on identifying signs of bleeding and trace it over the whole body including urine and stool (e.g. , petechial, mucosal bleeding, soft tissue bleeding, ecchymosis), as well as signs of systemic disease, for example, jaundice, and the size of liver and spleen should be noted. The presence of concomitant illness can be an indication for the cause of bleeding.

Petechial bleeding is usually presented in primary hemostatic disorders, especially thrombocytopenia or thrombocytopathy. Other signs of primary hemostatic disorders are small, and/or many scattered ecchymoses, as well as mucosal hemorrhages. Ecchymosis, large bruises or palpable hematomas in unusual places may suggest both primary and secondary bleeding disorders. When there is epistaxis, the nose should be examined to exclude excoriations and damaged vessels as the results of trauma. Joint and intramuscular bleeding with or without trauma is always abnormal in children and suggestive for especially secondary bleeding disorders.

（4）重点语句

Leukemia

Can I have a look on the blood spots?

Is there any other place where you notice irregular bleeding?

Do you feel bone or joint pain?

Do you have a fever?

Did someone from your family suffer from similar condition?

Have you had some medicine recently?

Anemia

Do you feel more tired than usual?

Have you noticed any change in your stool?

Did you have any health problems before?

What about your periods?

6. 内 分 泌 科

（1）内分泌科常见症状 / 疾病：多饮、多食、体重下降 Polydipsia, Polyphagia and Weight Loss

Warming up

This was a patient with a chief complain about polydipsia, polyphagia and weight loss. These were the typical clinical features of diabetes mellitus (DM). And the differential diagnosis of DM was the thyroid diseases, tumors and other chronic diseases. The doctors should pay attention to the patients' clinical manifestations as well as their laboratory examinations.

History taking

D: Hello, my name is XX. Now I want to know more details about your disease. Please sit down and answer my questions.

P: OK.

D: What should I call you?

P: My name is Li Gang from Shanxi Province. I'm 50 years old.

D: What's troubling you?

P: I feel polydipsia and polyuria.

D: How long have you been like this?

P: More than fifteen years.

D: Were there any inducement?

P: No.

D: *Did you notice anything associated with when this trouble starts?*

P: My weight decreased.

D: *Did you go to see the doctor and test your blood glucose?*

P: Yes. With fasting blood glucose was 7~8mmol/L, I was diagnosed with diabetes mellitus in the local hospital and the doctor advice diet therapy.

D: *What about your blood glucose monitoring?*

P: At the beginning, blood glucose is not monitored and symptoms of polydipsia, polyuria and weight loss worsened 3~4 months later. Then I was treated by a kind of oral drugs called "Xiaokewan".

D: Did you use other drugs?

P: I took in phenformin and metformin.

D: What was the dose of them?

P: I didn't remember it.

D: ***What about the effects of these drugs?***

P: The blood glucose was controlled during normal range.

D: Did you change the drug use?

P: 10 years ago, Novolin 30R was used.

D: Why?

P: Considering the side effects of oral drugs in liver and kidney.

D: What was the dosage of it?

P: 8～10U in the morning and 12U in the evening by hypodermic injection.

D: What was the effect? What about your blood glucose level?

P: the fasting blood glucose was 7～8mmol/L and postprandial blood glucose was 14～17mmol/L.

D: ***Did you suffer from the side effect of Novolin 30R?***

P: palpitations and perspiration before the meal.

D: How many times did it happen every week?

P: I didn't remember.

D: How did you deal with the situation?

P: Novolin 30R pen insulin syringes were used and the hypoglycemia response happened less frequently.

D: OK. Have you changed your regimen then?

P: Yes. I changed my regimen then. The therapeutic regimen changed to insulin injection for 3～4months and phenformin, metformin or other oral drugs for 8～9 months.

D: **_Why did you change the regimen?_**

P: Given inconvenience of insulin injection.

D: Have you remembered the dosage?

P: No.

D: Were there some other symptoms happen after adjusting the regimen?

P: I felt numbness in both lower extremities and pinching pain occurred and then I was treated in the local hospital every year.

D: How can you release the numbness and pain?

P: Methycobal.

D: How did you use it?

P: By intramuscular and intravenous drip infusion and the symptoms got better.

D: Have you been to other hospitals and done some tests?

P: I was hospitalized in PUMCH in December, 2011 and was diagnosed with type 2 diabetes mellitus with glycosylated hemoglobin 8.2% and fasting blood glucose 6.7mmol/L.

D: What was your treatment and how did you use the drugs?

P: Lantus 12U by hypodermic injection before sleep and Glucobay one pill once, three times a day.

D: How about the effect of treatment?

P: Fasting blood glucose among 4～6mmol/L and postprandial blood glucose among 6～11mmol/L.

D: What was your blood glucose level after you discharged?

P: The blood glucose was controlled poorly with fasting blood glucose 6～9mmol/L and postprandial blood glucose 15～17mmol/L.

D: Anything else?

P: Hypoglycemia happened many times at night at the lowest level 2.8mmol/L.

D: What did you do then? Did you ask for help to the doctor?

P: The patient was hospitalized again on Mar 18th, 2014 with fasting blood glucose 11.7mmol/L, 2h-plasma glucose 13.0mmol/L.

D: Did you do some tests?

P: Yes. The tests I did in the hospital are in the paper. (TC 4.31mmol/L, TG 2.23mmol/L, HDL-C 0.77mmol/L, LDL-C 2.66mmol/L, glycosylated hemoglobin 8.3%, ACR 0.08mg/mmolCr, thyroid function normal).

D: What about your symptoms?

P: Be worse. Compared to the condition in December, 2011, I lost 6kg and felt chest congestion.

D: When did chest congestion happen?

P: After minor activities.

D: How did you relieve the chest congestion?

P: After rest. But sometimes chest congestion occurred at rest and alleviated itself in minutes.

D: What about your eyesight?

P: Vision was impaired.

D: Are there other symptoms occurred recently?

P: Weakness of both lower extremities also occurred.

D: What about your diet and rest?

P: I eat staple 2～4 tael every meal and have much meat if I want to. I don't exercise in daily life.

D: What about your stool, urine and nocturia?

P: I have dry stool once per day and urine with foam, nocturia twice per night.

D: Do you have chronic disease such as hypertension, liver disease and kidney disease?

P: No.

D: Did you hurt or have operation?

P: No.

D: Are you allergic to special food or drugs?

P: No.

D: Have you been to the epidemic area?

P: No. I was born and living in Shanxi Province.

D: What's your occupation?

P: I am a salesman.

D: Do you smoke or addict to alcohol?

P: I smoke more than 40 years, 20～60 cigarettes every day and alcohol use more than 30 years, 5～6 tael every day.

D: Could you tell me about your marriage?

P: I am married and have a son. My wife and my son were both in good state of health.

D: Is there any history of diabetes in your family?

P: My parents and two brothers suffered from the same disease.

After examination done...

D: Having examined you, according to the guideline, you are diagnosed with diabetes mellitus. Diabetes is a kind of microangiopathy that involves many systems, especially eye, kidney and peripheral nerves. So the symptoms newly happened are chronic complications associated with diabetes, which is the primary disease.

I'm going to have you admitted to the ward right away so that your treatment can start at once. We'll start you on medication to decrease the blood glucose level and keep the level stable. I expect you'll have more examination to evaluate your various systems.

It's important that you need to have low sugar diet and exercise properly also.

I expect the treatment will improve your feeling. However, you may not get rid of it completely. We can never be absolutely certain about the future but you should remain optimistic. Do you have any question?

（2）内分泌科常见症状 / 疾病：甲状腺肿 Thyroid Swelling (Goiter)

Warm up

The problems facing the clinician, when confronted by a patient with a nodular goiter or thyroid nodule, are to determine whether the lesion is symptomatic, and whether it is benign or malignant. The differential diagnoses include benign goiter, intrathyroidal cysts, thyroiditis, benign, malignant tumors, and metastatic tumours to the thyroid. The history should specifically emphasize the duration of swelling, recent growth, local symptoms (dysphagia, pain, or voice changes), and systemic symptoms (hyperthyroidism, hypothyroidism, or those from possible tumours metastatic to the thyroid). The patient's age, sex, place of birth, family history, and history of radiation to the neck, are important.

The clinician must systematically palpate the thyroid to determine whether there is a solitary thyroid nodule or if it is a multinodular gland, and whether there are palpable lymph nodes. A solitary hard thyroid nodule is likely to be malignant, whereas most multinodular goiters are benign. Ultrasound evaluation helps document the number of nodules, whether a nodule is suspicious for cancer, and whether there are coexistent suspicious lymph nodes. In many patients, the possibility of cancer is difficult to exclude without microscopic examination of the gland itself, by percutaneous needle biopsy. Radioiodine thyroid scanning is used selectively to determine whether a follicular neoplasm by cytologic examination is functioning (warm or hot) or nonfunctioning (cold). A chest x-ray including the neck helps in demonstrating tracheal displacement, any calcification of the thyroid nodule, or the presence of pulmonary metastases. CT or MRI are usually not required but are helpful when the limits of the tumour cannot be defined.

The main indications for surgical removal of a nodular goiter are: suspicion of or documented cancer, symptoms of pressure, hyperthyroidism, substernal extension, and cosmetic deformity.

History taking

P: Good morning, Dr. Wang!

D: Good morning, Mr. Zhang! What brings you here today?

P: I have noticed swelling in my neck while I was shaving.

D: Ah, when did you notice this swelling?

P: It's been a while. I think about 3～4 weeks. I didn't pay much attention to it.

D: Tell me more about it. *Is it increasing in size?*

P: Yes. I think that it has increased in size. It is unpleasant and unsightly to have a swelling on the front of my neck.

D: Does it ache? *Do you have any difficulty when you swallow liquid or solids?*

P: No, I don't any difficulty in eating or drinking. The swelling does not ache at all.

D: Did you notice any change in your voice?

P: No, I have not had any change in voice. I had a bad sore throat about 1 month back but it didn't affect my voice much.

D: How about any change in weight? Did you notice your clothes got a bit loose or tight?

P: Not really. I wear pretty much the same size of clothes as before and they all fit me well.

D: Do you feel your heart pounding at times, especially at rest? (Do you get palpitations?)

P: No. I haven't noticed something like that so far. I do feel my heart thumping when I get busy with a lot of work or when I complete my jogging rounds every Friday!

D: How about any change in bowel habits lately? *Have you experienced any episodes of loose motions or constipation?*

P: Ah, I can recall I had loose bowl movements last week after I ate some food outside. It didn't last long though. I took two days off from work.

D: Well, may I examine you? If you are ready, please sit on the couch in front.

P: What am I supposed to do Dr. Wang? Shall I take

off my scarf?

D: Yes please. Make yourself comfortable! *I will require you to swallow some water from a glass as I examine your neck swelling.*

P: Alright, Doctor! I am ready for the examination.

D: After having examined you, I have to confirm that you indeed have a nodular swelling in your thyroid gland.

P: Oh! Is that very serious doctor? What is the treatment for this?

D: Well, to confirm the nature of this swelling, I suggest that we begin with some blood tests like thyroid function test, an ultrasound of your neck, a thyroid scintigraphy scan and to complement all of them with a fine needle aspiration cytology. Let's get started with the blood tests first!

P: Alright then! I believe I am in safe hands in here. Would that mean that I will end up requiring surgery? What is fine needle aspiration cytology? Does it hurt?

D: You'll be fine. The fine needle aspiration is usually carried under ultrasound guidance to harvest cells from the nodular swelling lesion, which are then viewed under the microscope. Depending on all your tests, we will then come to a diagnosis and afterwards we can formulate the treatment regimen. Surgery is usually advised under certain specific situations which I will explain to you if that is necessary course.

（3）内分泌科重点查体

Assessment of thyroid status

General inspection thin, anxious, sweaty, flushed, restless (hyper-)

Overweight, dry hair, croaky voice (hypo-)

Face proptosis, exophthalmos, lid retraction/lag (hyper-)

Coarse features, periorbital skin oedema (hypo-)

Loss of hair in lateral third of eyebrows (hypo-)

Malar flush (hypo-)

Hands hot sweaty palms, palmar eryfhema (hyper-)

Cold, dry hands (hypo-)

Radial pulse, tachycardia and bounding pulse, afrial fibrillafion (hyper-)

Bradycardia (hypo-)

Proximal muscle weakness of pectoral and pelvic girdle (hyper-) supinator and ankle jerks for delayed relaxation (hypo-)

（4）重点语句

Did you notice anything associated with when this trouble starts?

What about your blood glucose monitoring?

What was your treatment and how did you use the drugs?

Did you suffer from the side effect of Novolin 30R?

Why did you change the regimen?

What about your stool, urine and nocturia?

Are there other symptoms occurred recently?

Do you smoke or addict to alcohol?

Is it increasing in size?

Do you have any difficulty when you swallow liquid or solids?

Have you experienced any episodes of loose motions or constipation?

I will require you to swallow some water from a glass as I examine your neck swelling.

7. 风湿免疫科

（1）风湿免疫科常见症状 / 疾病：关节痛 Arthralgia

Warming up

Arthralgia, which is mostly defined as pain of the joints but can also be accompanied by articular swelling, is one of the most common symptoms seen in rheumatic diseases, including connective diseases such as rheumatoid arthritis (RA), systemic lupus erythematosus (SLE), spondyloarthropathy, osteoarthritis, and crystal arthropathies like gouty arthritis. Different patterns of arthralgia exist and indicate the underlying causes. Moreover, many other situations, including injury, tumor and infection, etc. Beside sterile inflammatory conditions may also lead to the presentation of arthralgia.

The history taking should at least include the following aspects: sites and number of joints involved, duration of each onset and time span of the whole disease, exacerbating and relieving factors, associated symptoms (especially extra-articular ones), intensity and nature of the pain (sharp or dull). Also, personal details, such as age, gender, occupation, as well as family history, can be useful clues for diagnosis.

History taking

D: Hello, what can I do for you?

P: I have pain in my knees and wrists. Several of my

knuckles feel tender to the touch as well.

D: When did you first notice the symptoms?

P: At least 2 months ago and things are not relieving.

D: *Does your pain move around?*

P: No, it's kind of restricted and will never fully go away once happens.

D: Is the pain sharp or dull?

P: Dull, I think. I can bear it most of the time.

D: *Is the pain always the same and persistent during the whole day?*

P: Actually not. The hardest time is during the morning after my waking up but it feels better within 2 hours.

D: *Do you have stiffness with your joints?*

P: Yes, especially with my fingers. It's more obvious in the morning as well.

D: *Are there any swelling joint?*

P: Yes, my joints seem swollen a lot.

D: *Do you feel any decline in the movement range of your joints?*

P: Yes, I can't stretch my fingers and legs as much as I could before.

D: *Have you experienced fatigue or a rise of body temperature?*

P: Yes, sometimes I feel like resting more than I used to, and the body temperature could be up to 37.5℃.

D: Do you cough a lot?

P: Not really.

D: Have you noticed any rashes?

P: No.

D: Have you ever done anything or taken any

medication to relieve the pain?

P: I tried taking some ibuprofen at home. It helped a little but the pain came back once I stopped the medication.

D: Is this your first time to come to hospital because of your joint pain?

P: No, I've visited the local hospital and done some basic blood tests. Here are the results.

D: These tests show that you have mild anemia, and the inflammation in your body is more active than normal. I need to examine your joints and other parts of your body. Would you mind lying on the examination bed please? ... I suggest we do an ultrasound test to assess the situation of your joints and some more blood tests that could help with the diagnosis.

Communication and interpretation

D: It is highly possible that you have rheumatic arthritis, which means that some of your joints are attacked by your own immune cells. It could explain the discomfort of your knees, wrists and fingers, your fatigue and those abnormal results of your blood tests.

P: How did I get this disease? Is the inflammation caused by some kind of infection? Is the disease going to progress?

D: The mechanism of the disease could be quite complicated. In general, the inflammation is directed toward your own body other than viruses or bacteria. However, the exact causes remained unclear. Without proper treatment, rheumatoid arthritis patients could eventually have their joints dislocated and deformed, but we've got several options for you to control the symptoms and prevent the disease from developing further. What else would you like to know?

P: Nothing more. Thanks for your help.

（2）风湿免疫科常见症状 / 疾病：系统性红斑狼疮 Systemic Lupus Erythematosus（SLE）

Warming up

SLE is a typical connective tissue disease characterized by involvement of multiple systems. Varied manifestations and severity might be observed in different individuals, requiring physicians to capture the whole script rather than focus on certain minor symptoms. When presented with cases showing signs, clinicians should explore the disease history thoroughly in order to determine the likely diagnosis and exclude other underlying causes. Symptoms can be grouped as following:

1) Systemic symptoms: fever, fatigue, etc.

2) Musculoskeletal symptoms: muscle weakness, arthritis, etc.

3) Skin-mucosal symptoms: rashes (malar rash, discord rash, ect), mouth ulcers, photosensitivity, hair loss, etc.

4) Cardiovascular symptoms: Raynaud's phenomenon, chest tightness, palpitation, etc.

5) Upper respiratory symptoms: epistaxis, etc.

6) Lower respiratory symptoms: cough, chest pain, dyspnea, etc.

7) Gastrointestinal symptoms: dysphagia, stomachache, etc.

8) Renal symptoms: hematuria, proteinuria, etc.

9) Hematologic symptoms: fatigue, shortness of breath, epistaxis, bleeding gums, etc.

10) Neuropsychiatric symptoms: headache, numb, seizures, psychosis, etc.

11) Other symptoms: dry eyes, recurrent miscarriage, etc.

It should be noted that the history taking is supposed to be well-oriented based on the known symptoms instead of aimless questioning.

History taking

D: Hello, how may I help you?

P: I'm having a fever. It's been a week.

D: What's your highest body temperature?

P: 38.3℃.

D: When does it usually peak, during the day or night?

P: I'm not very sure about this but I think I feel worse in the afternoon.

D: Do you cough or anything?

P: No, it seems strange because I'm not coughing, sneezing, having a runny nose, sore throat, or headache.

D: Is there any pain in your joints or muscles?

P: Yes, my joints have been sometimes painful since the fever, but the pain moves around.

D: *Have you ever noticed the rashes on your cheeks?*

P: Yes, they appeared about 1 month ago and worsen on sunny days. I thought I might have an allergy toward the cosmetics so I didn't go to the clinic.

D: Have your had other rashes?

P: I haven't noticed anymore yet.

D: *Have you had any mouth ulcers?*

P: No.

D: *Is there any hair loss?*

P: Yes, it has been really obvious the past few days.

D: *Do you have trouble with lifting things or standing up after sitting?*

P: I tend to get exhausted these days, but it wasn't that severe until recently.

D: *Is there any change of color or increased foam in the urine?*

P: It does seem a little foamy.

D: Do you have swollen legs, ankles, feet or face?

P: Yes, I think so.

D: Do you have chest pain?

P: No.

D: Have you experience any emotional fluctuation?

P: No, I don't think there is any change in my emotional behavior.

D: Is there any hearing or vision loss?

P: No.

D: Do you have a stomachache?

P: No.

D: How is your stool?

P: It's just as usual.

D: Is this the first time you come to a hospital since these symptoms began?

P: No, I got my blood tested yesterday and here are the reports.

D: It appears that there is some blood cell destruction in your body. Large amounts of protein were found in your urine specimen. We might need further tests to determine your diagnosis and treatment plan. Before that, can I examine you please?......

Communication and interpretation

D: Considering the symptoms you have now and the tests result available, I think you may have the disease called systemic lupus erythematosus. This is a variety of disease that might be caused by the imbalance of your immune system.

P: Do you mean that my fever was not caused by infection?

D: Probably not. To support our diagnosis, we'd like to do several more blood tests, which can show the level of the immune responses within your body. Besides, we need to quantify the amount of the protein in your urine. I'm also going to arrange a chest X-ray, an ECG, an echocardiography, and a renal biopsy examination.

P: I don't feel like doing the biopsy thing. It sounds terrible.

D: The biopsy examination is of great importance to the determination of your diagnosis and therapy. It can also help us predicting your response to treatment.

We highly recommend that you go through the examination.

P: Alright then. Is my situation quite severe?

D: Lupus can damage several organs. Some of the damage can be tough to handle with, so it's crucial to receive effective and regular medication. As I have explained, the disease is resulted from the immune dysfunction, so some drugs aimed to regulate your immune function will help with your recover. Do you have any other questions?

P: No, thank you.

（3）风湿免疫科重点查体

1) peripheral and axial joints

Swelling: Severe joint swelling can be noticed by inspection and is often seen with regional redness, indicating local inflammation. Floating patella test positive indicates the volume of the synovial fluid in the articular cavity is over 50ml.

Tenderness: Joint tenderness is another hallmark of reginal inflammation. In spondyloarthropathy, Patrick sign suggests sacroiliitis and consistent body signs might be found when enthesitis is present.

Range of motion: Loss of mobility can be permanent. Caused by bone, cartilage, or tendon damage. Reversible case are usually resulted from active inflammation.

Deformity: Some forms of articular deformity are of high diagnostic value and often imply a late disease phase, like swan neck deformity and boutonniere deformity in rheumatoid arthritis, Bouchard and Heberden nodule in osteoarthritis and gout stone in gouty arthritis.

2) Skin and mucosa

Some rashes are specific to a certain disease. For example, malar rash is unique to SLE and heliotrope rash indicates dermatomyositis. Other skin lesions are non-specific but should also be noted, like mouth ulcers in Sjogren syndrome, SLE, Behcet's disease, and livedo reticularis in several rheumatoid diseases.

（4）重点语句

Arthralgia

Does your pain move around?

Is the pain always the same and persistent during the whole day?

Do you have stiffness with your joints?

Do you feel any decline in the movement range of your joints?

Have you experienced fatigue or a rise of body temperature?

Systemic lupus erythematosus

Have you ever noticed rashes on your cheeks?

Have you had any ulcers, mouth or others?

Is there any hair loss?

Do you have trouble with lifting things or standing up after sitting?

Is there any change in color or increased foam in the urine?

8. 神 经 内 科

（1）神经内科常见症状 / 疾病：缺血性卒中 Ischemia Stroke

Warming up

A stroke is the loss of brain function due to a disturbance in the blood supply to the brain. Stroke (ischemia and hemorrhagic) is the second leading cause death of the world and is one of the leading causes of adult disability. Overall, approximately 80% of strokes are ischemic stroke. The definition of ischemic stroke is brain, spinal cord, or retinal cell death due to ischemia with neuropathologic, neuroimaging, or clinical evidence of permanent injury.

Ischemic stroke is a medical emergency and can cause permanent neurological damage or death. Risk factors for ischemic stroke include old age, high blood pressure, previous stroke or transient ischemic attack (TIA), diabetes, high cholesterol, tobacco smoking, and atrial fibrillation. High blood pressure is the most important modifiable risk factor of ischemic stroke. According to the severity and situation, choice of treatments are different including drug therapy and surgery. Treatment to recover any lost function is termed stroke rehabilitation. Ideally, this would take place in a stroke unit and involving health professions such as speech and language therapy, physical therapy and occupational therapy.

History taking

D: Hi. What brought you to the hospital this time?

P: I lost consciousness suddenly this morning.

D: Oh, when did it happen and what were you doing at that time?

P: Around 7 o'clock in the morning while I was making breakfast.

D: Do you know what happened after that?

P: I passed out and I don't know what happened. My wife said she saw me slide down by the cabinet. She ran over to help me while I sat on the ground.

D: *How long were you unconscious?*

P: My wife and I are not so sure about that. She was

scared. I guess it lasted for about 10 minutes.

D: Did your wife see any other signs or symptoms after you passed out, such as body twitches, shakes (convulsions), or foaming at the mouth?

P: My wife said no.

D: *Do you have any other unusual feelings, such as headache or nausea?*

P: No.

D: *Do you have any trouble on walking, feel any dizziness, lack of balance, or coordination?*

P: Well, I am still a little dizzy.

D: *Is there numbness or weakness of the face, arms, or legs, especially on one side of the body?*

P: Yes, my right hand is a little numb and it feels weak.

D: *Did you have any trouble in speaking or understanding other people's speech?*

P: No.

D: *Have you ever experienced this situation before?*

P: I've had similar dizziness episodes 3 times in the past but did not lose consciousness. I also have numbness on hands and arms, occasionally.

D: *When did these symptoms start?*

P: About one year ago.

D: Did you ever see a doctor or go to the emergency room for that?

P: Never. I did not know it was a serious problem at that time. I thought I just needed to take a break.

D: *Do you have any other medical problems, such as high blood pressure, heart disease, or other problems?*

P: I have high blood pressure and diabetes.

D: Do you take any medications?

P: I take 1 tablet of nifedipine per day and 1 tablet of metformin before meals.

D: What does your blood pressure and blood sugar levels like at home?

P: My blood pressure is usually 160/110mmHg and my blood sugar is around 7～8mmol/L.

D: Got it. How is your family's health? Especially your parents. Are they still alive? Did they have any significant medical problems or have similar complaints?

P: My father has a history of high blood pressure, and my mother died of cerebra infarction.

D: Do you smoke?

P: Yes, but not so much. About 10 cigarettes per day.

D: OK, now could you lie down in the bed for me; if it is okay with you, I will go ahead and do a quick exam.

D: Thank you. You can sit up now. I think the next step would be a CT examination to help clarify the diagnosis. After my assessment and exam, I recommend that you be admitted to the hospital for further workup and treatment.

Communication and interpretation

D: After physical examination and CT scan, I think you are suffering from a transient ischemia attack (TIA), which is a brief episode of neurologic dysfunction resulting from focal cerebral ischemia with no evidence of corresponding tissue injury. Next step, to clear the condition I will arrange for you to perform a cerebral angiography for the cerebral vascular related information with CTA or MRA. Digital subtraction angiography is the most accurate method for diagnosis of the disease; however, the harm and costs are relatively larger than CTA or MRA.

P: Doctor, is it that bad? What are the next step for treatment?

D: Please don't worry at this stage. Currently, diagnostic evaluation and treatment options of these diseases have become more mature, and early detection, early diagnosis, and early treatment has improved prognosis for most patients.

For treatment, depending on the severity and situation, we can choose different options including drug therapy and surgery. If there is no obvious cerebrovascular stenosis, we will give you drug therapy such as antiplatelets and antihypertensives. But there is obvious cerebral arterial stenosis, surgery may need to be done. Of course, you will need to aggressively treat your high blood pressure and diabetes. Lifestyle adjustments, such as eating healthy foods and quitting smoking, may reduce the risk of stroke. Do you have any question?

P: No. I got it. Thank you very much.

（2）神经内科常见症状 / 疾病：出血性卒中 Hemorrhagic Stroke

Warming up

About 20% of all strokes are attributed to spontaneous intracranial hemorrhage. Spontaneous intracranial hemorrhage includes intracerebral hemorrhages (approximately three quarters) and subarachnoid hemorrhages (approximately one quarter).

Intracerebral hemorrhages mainly result from the rupture of small penetrating arteries. However, subarachnoid hemorrhages often result from a rupture of vessels on the brain's surface due to a congenital aneurysm. So hemorrhagic stroke leads to blood entering directly into the brain parenchyma or into the subarachnoid space surrounding brain tissue. Additionally, both types of hemorrhagic stroke have high mortality rates, but recovery and survival have improved in recent decades due to advances in neurocritical care.

Cigarete smoking, heavy alcohol use, chronic and poorly controlled hypertension, and use of sympathomimetic agents are modifiable risk factors for subarachnoid hemorrhage. Compared with no therapy, the use of warfarin, especially the international normalized ratio (INR) is higher than 3, but not of aspirin is associated with an increased risk of intracerebral hemorrhage. So, hemorrhagic strokes are preventable to some degree.

History taking

D: Hello! How may I help you?

P: Doctor, I have a severe "thunderclap" headache.

D: *When did the symptom begin?*

P: One hour ago.

D: What were you doing at that time?

P : I was on the toilet. I was pushing hard because I was constipated.

D: *Do you have any other uncomfortable symptom such as stiff neck, nausea, or vomiting?*

P: Yes, I have some neck pain and nausea, but have not vomited.

D: Did you lose consciousness?

P: No.

D: *Is there any numbness or tingling of the face, arms, or legs, especially just one side of your body?*

P: No, I don't feel any of that.

D: *Did you have any trouble in speaking or understanding other people's speech?*

P: No.

D: *Are there any changes in vision, such as loss of vision?*

P: No, but I could not see for a while when the headache occurred.

D: Have you ever experienced this situation before?

P: In the past several weeks, I have headaches several times, but not as severe as this time. This really is the worst headache I have ever had!

D: How long have you had these headaches?

P: About a month and a half.

D: Did you ever see a doctor or go to the emergency room for that?

P: No, I did not take it as serious problem and I thought I was catching a cold.

D: Have you had any medical conditions in the past?

P: No, I am not aware of any medical problems. I hardly ever take any medications.

D: *How is your family's health? Do they have any significant medical problems or have similar complaints?*

P: My parents are healthy, but my little brother died nine years ago because of cerebral hemorrhage. Is this disease genetic?

D: I am not sure about that since I don't know the exact details of your brother's situation. Do you smoke?

P: No.

D: What about alcohol?

P: I drink occasionally, but not too much.

D: OK good. Next step, I'm going to do a quick physical exam for you. To help clarify the diagnosis, I think you may need a CT scan. After my assessment and results from the imaging study, I think you need to be admitted to the hospital for further monitoring and treatment.

Communication and interpretation

D: Based on my assessment and results from the imaging study, I think you are suffering from a subarachnoid hemorrhage. The most common cause of a subarachnoid hemorrhage is the rupture of vessels on the brain's surface due to a congenital aneurysm, which may occur at any age but is most common from age 40 to 65. Additionally, according to the clinical data, women are more likely to suffer from it than men. When a subarachnoid hemorrhage occurs, a person may experience a rapidly developing, severe "thunderclap" headache and other commonly associated symptoms including stiff neck, loss of consciousness, nausea, vomiting, back or leg pain, and photophobia.

P: Oh, that sounds terrible! What should I do now?

D: Subarachnoid hemorrhages are a type of hemorrhagic stroke and have high mortality rates, but recovery and survival have improved in recent decades due to advances in neurocritical care. So, I recommend that you be admitted to the hospital so that your treatment can start at once.

Firstly, to find out if there are any ruptured aneurysms, you may need a brain angiography with CTA or MRA. Digital subtraction angiography is the most accurate method for diagnosis of the disease currently. Additionally, you may also need an electrocardiogram (EKG) to evaluate the dramatic stress on the brain.

For treatment, we will give you medication to relieve the symptoms and prevent complications such as permanent brain damage. If the hemorrhage is due to an aneurysm rupture, then surgery is needed. If no aneurysm is found, you will be closely monitored and may need more imaging tests in 2 weeks. During this time, you may need to be on strict bed rest. You will be given medication to prevent seizures and control blood pressure. Additionally, some pain medications and anti-anxiety pills are also needed. Is there anything that you wish to ask?

P: No. I got it. Thank you very much.

（3）神经内科重点查体

1) Assessing the higher mental function

During a careful medical history in stroke patients, assessment of mental status is needed to adequately assess the level of consciousness, orientation, memory, language function, affect, and judgment.

2) Assessing the cranial nerves

When a stroke occurs, a cranial nerve function test includes visual acuity (with and without correction), optic fundi, visual fields, pupils (size and reactivity to direct and consensual light), ocular motility, jaw, facial, palatal, neck, tongue movement, and hearing.

3) Assessing the peripheral nervous system

Motor system: Assessment of the motor system is essential in all stroke patients including muscle tone (flaccid, spastic or rigid), muscle size (atrophy or hypertrophy), and muscle power. Assessing the motor system in the upper and lower limbs, both proximally and distally, and comparing one muscle group with the same group on the other side, are essential.

Sensation: Sensory testing need not be detailed if there are no sensory symptoms in stroke patients. However, vibration perception in the toes and the normality of perception of pain, temperature, and light touch in the hands and feet should be assessed by evaluating right-left comparison.

Reflexes: Muscle stretch reflexes and plantar responses should always be assessed by evaluating right-left symmetry and disparity between proximal and distal reflexes or arm and leg reflexes. Biceps, triceps, brachioradialis, quadriceps, and ankle reflexes should be quantitated from 1 to 4 (4 = clonus; 3 = spread; 2 = brisk; 1 = hypoactive).

（4）重点语句

Ischemia stroke

How long were you unconscious?

Do you have any other unusual feelings, such as headache or nausea?

Do you have any trouble walking or any dizziness, lack of balance, or coordination?

Is there numbness or weakness of the face, arms, or legs, especially on one side of the body?

Did you have any trouble in speaking or understanding other people's speech?

Have you ever experienced this situation before?

When did these symptoms start?

Do you have any other medical problems, such as high blood pressure, heart disease, or other problems?

Hemorrhagic stroke

When did the symptoms begin?

Do you have any other uncomfortable symptoms, such as stiff neck, nausea, or vomiting?

Is there any numbness or tingling of face, arms, or legs, especially just one side of your body?

Did you have any trouble in speaking or understanding other people's speech?

Is there any changes in vision, such as loss of vision?

How is your family's health? Did they have any significant medical problems or have similar complaints?

9. 骨　　科

（1）骨科常见症状 / 疾病：骨折 Fracture

Warming up

A fracture refers to complete or incomplete break of bone continuity due to external force. In young and healthy people, fractures usually happen after a comparatively high energy impact on skeletal system. However, in the elderly, fractures may occur easily in osteoporotic bones after a mild injury. Among them, femoral neck and distal radius are the two crispest sites, especially in elderly women. Sometimes they may occur together after a typical fall.

Plain X-rays are usually enough for diagnosis of fracture. CT and MRI are more helpful for further assessment of fracture classification. Conservative treatment is routinely applied on stable fractures which can be fixed with a plaster after reduction. However, internal fixation after open reduction can be more suitable for comminuted, complicated, and intra-articular fractures. Femoral neck fractures may lead to avascular necrosis of femoral head. Therefore, hip joint replacement surgery is the best option for elderly patients.

Rehabilitation plays an important role in function recovery after fracture. Patients are always encouraged to exercise their joints and muscles after plaster fixation or surgery.

History taking

D: Good morning, madam. What's the matter? How can I help?

P: Good morning, doctor! *It's so bad! I hurt myself just one hour ago.* It feels quite painful on my buttock and hands now.

D: Oh, how did it happen?

P: I fell down suddenly while I was walking along the street early this morning. I'm afraid I didn't notice an obstacle in front of my feet.

D: Do you mean that it was an accident?

P: I think so. *I tried to support my body with my hands the moment I lost my balance.* However, I failed and then fell on the ground. I was not able to stand up again.

D: I see. Did you lose consciousness at that moment?

P: Absolutely not. I called "911" by myself. That's why I am in the emergency room now.

D: Hmm, that's clear. By the way, do you often fall down?

P: Well, sometimes. Both my knees are not good enough especially when I walk upstairs and downstairs. I remember I got patella fracture in my left knee some years ago, which was also due to a fall. Fortunately I recovered well.

D: OK. ***Do you hurt anywhere else this morning?*** I mean, your head, chest, or back for example?

P: No, I don't think so.

D: Do you have any chronic diseases in the past, such as hypertension, diabetes, or stroke?

P: I have been suffered from diabetes for many years. However, the glucose level is well controlled by oral diabetic drugs. Hypertension is not serious. No stroke in history.

D: How old are you? Have you checked your bone density before?

P: Ah yes, I remember I took such an examination two years ago, when I was 75 years old. The doctor said that the quality of my bone was not good and then prescribed me some medicine. I do have pain in my bones and joints sometimes.

D: You know, we call it osteoporosis. ***There will be a risk of fracture in porotic bones.*** Well, let me take a look at your injured limbs now. Please lie down on your back.

P: Oh, it seems to be difficult to lie down. It's really painful here.

D: No worry, it's OK. Your right lower limb is

externally rotated. It is about 1 cm shorter than the other side. Let me touch your buttock. No bruising but obvious pain and tenderness here. Actually it is not on the buttock, but the hip joint. ***Can you move it as you wish?***

P: No, doctor. I'm afraid I can't. It's almost impossible!

D: I think there might be a fracture within or around your hip joint. ***Hip fractures are quite common in women at your age.***

P: Oh, God! How about my hand? You see, it's so swollen.

D: I think you actually hurt your wrist instead of your hand. That's another site where fracture happens commonly in the elderly. ***I believe your wrist has been fractured, just according to the typical "dinner fork" deformity I can see.*** Now can you move your fingers?

P: Yes, I can but much more painful on my wrist.

D: That means your palm and fingers are not involved. Don't worry. Fractures can be treated properly in our hospital. Now I will send you to the radiology department to take some X-rays for confirmation.

Communication and interpretation

D: Hi, madam. The X-rays are available now. You fractured your hip and wrist joint. Specifically, it is a femoral neck fracture(Figure 2-1 & Figure 2-2) and a distal radius fracture(Figure 2-3 & Figure 2-4), both on the right side.

P: That's too bad! Do I need surgery? I am so nervous, you know.

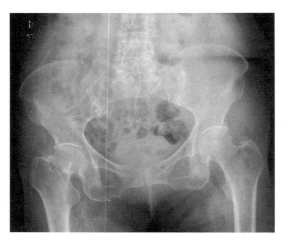

Figure 2-1 pelvis X-ray (AP view) of right femoral neck fracture

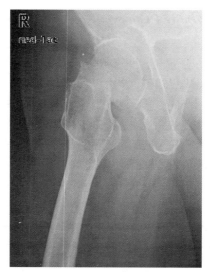

Figure 2-2 hip X-ray (lateral view) of right femoral neck fracture

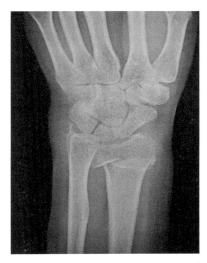

Figure 2-3 wrist X-ray (AP view) of right distal radius fracture

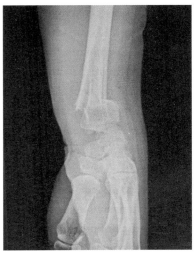

Figure 2-4 wrist X-ray (lateral view) of right distal radius fracture

D: Well, judging from the X-rays, *I think your wrist fracture can be treated conservatively.* Although it was displaced, the joint surface was not involved. If the fracture can be well reduced, plaster fixation for about six weeks is enough.

P: Really? Operation is not necessary?

D: Right. Most of distal radius fractures can be treated non-operatively unless the fracture is either intra-articular comminuted or in a special type leading to instability.

P: That's good! What about the hip joint?

D: I'm afraid you are not lucky enough in the fracture of femoral neck. *The femoral head was displaced posteriorly and inferiorly, indicating a very unstable fracture in the hip joint.*

P: So it needs an operation, I guess. Will you use some screws to fix it?

D: Internal fixation with screws might not be helpful in such a special fracture. This is because of a complication called avascular necrosis often occurs in femoral head even when it is well fixed during operation. In your case, most likely it would fail sooner or later.

P: It's that serious? What can be done then?

D: The option now is hip joint replacement. The femoral head will be removed first and then replaced with an artificial ball on a metal stem.

P: Oh, that's a big operation isn't it?

D: Not really. Hip joint replacement surgery is a regular operation now. The advantage is that you can walk on the next day after operation.

P: Sounds great though I still worry about the

treatment.

D: No worry! Let's deal with the wrist fracture first. See you soon in plaster room.

Half an hour later...

D: How do you feel inside the plaster? Is it uncomfortable?

P: Not as painful as before but it's a little bit heavy. It seems that my wrist is fixed in an uncomfortable position.

D: You will get used to it soon. ***Remember to flex and extend your thumb and fingers from time to time.***

P: OK, I will do. Thank you, doctor.

D: It's my pleasure. The nurse will make further arrangement for your admission. You will finish a preoperative assessment in the ward and then wait for surgery.

（2）骨科重点查体

1) Inspection

Swelling: It may confined to the joint, indicating excess synovial fluid, pus or blood in joint cavity; around the bone, indicating edema in soft tissue injury or hematoma due to fracture. In this case, swelling can be seen around distal radius. However, it cannot be noticed around the hip because the hematoma is deep in the hip joint cavity.

Bruising: It may suggest trauma, with a point of impact, gravitational, or other spread.

Deformity: It may occur in joint dislocation or fractures with obvious displacement. In this case, there might be a typical "dinner fork" or "bayonet" deformity due to dorsal and radial displacement of distal radius respectively. A completely displaced femoral neck fracture often leads to external rotation deformity of the whole lower limb.

Muscle wasting: It may occur as a result of disuse, pain, other incapacities, or from denervation of the muscles affected.

Shortening: It may occur in dislocation or displaced fractures. In femoral neck fracture with displacement, $1 \sim 2$cm shortening is common.

2) Palpation

Skin temperature: A localized increase in skin temperature generally indicates an inflammatory process in the underlying anatomical structure. Asymmetrical coldness of a limb occurs where limb circulation is impaired.

Tenderness: It may occur very commonly in any bone and joint trauma in limbs and spine, including fracture, dislocation, ligament, and other soft tissue injuries; occur in bone and joint inflammatory diseases such as acute osteomyelitis and septic arthritis. In this case, tenderness can be easily palpated at distal radius and femoral neck.

3) Movements

Joint movement: The movement of a joint normally includes flexion and extension. Some joints have abduction, adduction, internal rotation, external rotation and other special movement. Normal range of motion (ROM) varies in different joints. The limitation of movement may occur in dislocation or fractures especially when they are displaced or intra-articular.

Sometimes pain or other factors may restrict active movement to a range that is less than passive movement. In this case, the movement of wrist is largely restricted by displacement and deformity in distal radius. The loss of hip joint movement is due to displaced fracture in femoral neck.

Muscle strength: The strength of muscle contraction may be impaired by pain, waste from disuse, disease or denervation. It should be carefully assessed according to MRC scale ($M_0 \sim M_5$) when necessary.

4) Measurement

Range of motion: The angle of each movement of a joint can be measured with a protractor. Active and passive ROM should be measured respectively sometimes.

Length and perimeter: Length and perimeter of limbs are measured with a flexible ruler to see if there is any discrepancy due to shortening and muscle waste.

（3）重点语句

Fracture

It's so bad! I hurt myself just one hour ago.

I tried to support my body with my hands the moment I lost my balance.

Did you hurt anywhere else this morning?

There will be a risk of fracture in porotic bones.

Can you move it as you wish?

Hip fractures are quite common in women at your age.

I believe your wrist has been fractured, just according to the typical "dinner fork" deformity I can see.

I think your wrist fracture can be treated conservatively.

The femoral head was displaced posteriorly and inferiorly, indicating a very unstable fracture in the hip joint.

Remember to flex and extend your thumb and fingers from time to time.

10. 胸 心 外 科

（1）胸外科常见疾病：肺癌 Lung Cancer

Warming up

Lung cancer is the leading cause of cancer-related deaths among men and women worldwide. The signs and symptoms of lung cancer can take years to develop and they may not appear in advanced stages by the time of diagnosis. Based on treatment principle and prognosis, the bulk of patients can be divided into two major groups: non-small-cell lung cancer（NSCLC）, and small-cell lung caner（SCLC）. Early detection of lung cancer is important to improve survival. If the primary lung cancer has metastasized, a patient may feel symptoms in places other than chest in the body. Common places for lung cancer to spread include: other parts of lungs, pulmonary and mediastinal lymph nodes, bones, brain, liver, and adrenal glands. A careful history taking of the symptom or risk factors helps to diagnose lung cancer.

Symptoms of lung cancer:

1) Coughing, especially if it persists or becomes

intense

2) Coughing up blood or bloody phlegm

3) Being short of breath

4) Chest pain

5) Changes in the voice or being hoarse

6) Recurrent lung problems, such as bronchitis or pneumonia

7) Other general symptoms like weakness, fatigue, weight loss, headaches, bone or joint pain

Risk factors of lung cancer

1) Tobacco smoking

2) Contact with radon, asbestos or other cancer-causing agents

3) Having had certain other cancers

4) Family members who have had lung cancer

5) Having had other lung diseases

6) Contact with second-hand smoke

History taking

D: I am Dr. Ye, before we start, I just want to confirm your details, so it's Mr. Li Ming, 65 years old, and this is your address?

P: Yes, it's right.

D: *So how can I help you today?*

P: I have been coughing for several days, and my family doctor told me that I had a nodule in the left upper lobe of my lung on CT scan.

D: *And how long had this cough?*

P: Roughly one month.

D: *What color is your coughing up?*

P: Faint yellow.

D: *Have you coughed blood or bloody phlegm?*

P: Yes, sometimes.

D: Is it large amounts?

P: Not much.

D: ***Do you have any other breathing problems like shortness of breath or chest tightness?***

P: Not really.

D: Headaches or chest pain?

P: Not at all.

D: Do you smoke?

P: I do smoke.

D: How many cigarettes do you smoke in a day?

P: 2～3 packs a day.

D: How long have you smoked?

P: Since I was 20.

D: Have you ever thought about giving up smoking?

P: Not the moment.

D: Is there any chance you have been exposed to dust or any sort of radiation?

P: Barely any.

D: ***Do any members of your family have lung diseases?***

P: My uncle died of lung cancer.

D: Where is you CT film?

P: Here you are.

D: ***Well, I may need to examine you.***

Communication and interpretation

D: You can see there is a mass in the left upper lobe of your lung.

P: There is something in my lung? What is it?

D: It can be a number of things, it could be a benign tumor, a granuloma, an old tuberculosis lesion, it could be an inhaled foreign body, and it could be a lot of things. You have to undergo bronchoscopy, needle aspiration biopsy, or even exploratory surgery before we are sure. But I think you should regard it a potential serious finding.

P: What do you mean? You are saying it is lung cancer?

D: I am not saying that. I am saying we don't know anything for sure so far. Your history of coughing up bloody phlegm, history of heavy smoking and this chest CT scan is suggestive of lung cancer. But the diagnosis has not been confirmed and it might very well be something else, and none of us should jump to any conclusion until we know for sure. I suggest that you should be admitted for further evaluation.

P: Thank you doctor, I'll think it over.

（2）胸外科重点查体

1) General inspection: General patients should be evaluated according to the presenting of cachexia, cyanosis, coughing (dry or productive), respiratory rate (normally ranges from 12～20 breathe per minute), and signs of shortness of breath (tachypnea, tripod position, use of accessory muscles, flared nostrils). Horner's syndrome can be seen in Pancoast's tumor patient. Chest wall deformity (like "Barrel chest" in case of COPD), scars (previous drainage or surgical incision) and finger clubbing or cigarette staining should also be noticed.

2) Palpation: Careful checking for neck and

supraclavicular lymphadenopathy, trachea deviation (away from the side in tension pneumothorax and large pleural effusion. Towards to the side of collapsed lung or pneumonectomy). Chest expansion: unilaterally reduced when lung collapse or pneumonia.

3) Percussion: Dull percussion note when consolidation, lung collapse, pleural effusion exists. Hyperresonant when pneumothorax happens.

4) Auscultation: Inspiratory stridor can be heard when upper airway is obstructed and wheezing can be heard as air moves through a narrow airway, as in asthma and COPD. Coarse crackles are usually caused by mucus in the bronchi, as in obstructive pneumonia and fine crackles can be heard in patients with interstitial lung disease or pulmonary edema.

Vocal resonance: Ask the patient to say "99" during auscultation. Increased vocal resonance can be heard in case of consolidation, lobar collapse, and decreased vocal resonance in case of pleural effusion.

（3）重点语句

So how can I help you today?

And how long have you had this cough?

What color is your coughing up?

Have you coughed blood or bloody phlegm?

Do you have any other breathing problems like shortness of breath or chest tightness?

How many cigarettes do you smoke in a day?

Do any members of your family have lung diseases?

Well, I may need to examine you.

11. 神 经 外 科

（1）神经外科常见症状/疾病：头痛 Headache

Warming up

Headaches are defined as pain anywhere in the region of the head or neck. It is one of the most frequently encountered problems in daily general medical practice. About half of adults have a headache in a given year. The need for accurate diagnosis and proper treatment of a headache is beyond dispute. However, an accurate diagnosis in patients with headaches seems easy, but is actually quite difficult.

Headaches are classified as primary or secondary. Primary headaches is a syndrome unto themselves rather than sign of other diseases. Secondary headache is a symptom of other illnesses. Unlike primary headaches, secondary headaches are potentially dangerous.

The distinction of primary and secondary headache is useful diagnostically. Primary headache, such as tension headache, is diagnosed clinically. Secondary headache, such as headache caused by brain tumors, often can be definitively diagnosed by identifying the underlying disease.

History taking

D: Hello, how may I help you?

P: I have headache which is hurting more each day, so I thought I should come and see you.

D: *Is this headache new or old?*

P: It started about half a year ago.

D: *What kind of headache is it?*

P: It is a sharp and stabbing-like pain.

D: *How often does it occur?*

P: It occurs almost every day, especially this month.

D: *In which part of the head do you have the headache?*

P: Entire head.

D: *When do the headaches tend to occur?*

P: Mostly early morning.

D: *Do you take medicine regularly for the headaches?*

P: No, I am afraid of the side effects of the medication, so I usually just suffer the headaches.

D: *Do you have an aura, like a flickering or blind spot, in the visual field?*

P: No, I don't have any vision loss.

D: *Do you experience any abnormal vision?*

P: I sometimes have blurred vision with halos around lights.

D: *Do you experience nausea or vomiting?*

P: Yes. When the headache is severe, I suffer from nausea and vomiting.

D: *Do you feel depressed?*

P: No, I don't have any psychological symptoms.

D: *Does anyone in your family have headaches?*

P: No. My parents are healthy, they don't have headache history.

D: Do you take some medicine or have exposure to toxins before you had these headaches?

P: No. I didn't try something or change my lifestyle.

D: Let me have a look. I'd like to test your vision and visual fields firstly. Headaches are a very common symptom, which can be caused by a number of reasons, such as stress, drug use, infection, toxins, vascular disease, neurotic diseases, and sympathetic and functional reasons. I think we should do a brain MRI to help assess your condition.

Communication and interpretation

D: The MRI shows that you might have a space-occupying lesion, in other words, a tumor, in your brain. The lesion can cause the intracranial hypertension symptoms including headache, nausea and vomiting.

Headaches usually occur at night and in the morning, but more severe in the morning. Headache symptoms worsen during coughing, sneezing, and defecation. Vomiting is usually projectile vomiting, which afterwards will relieve headache.

This is generally not related to diet. Nerve compression causes reduced vision and defect of your visual field. At the late stage, you may have hemiplegia, which manifests one side of the body, single limb weakness, paralysis and hemianesthesia manifested by numbness of one limb, hypoalgesia, hypothermia, abnormal sensation, loss of depth perception, two-point discrimination, image sense, material sense and physical sense.

It may also cause personality changes. Some people become dull, lazy, have short-term memory loss or even long-term memory loss, serious loss of balance, lack of judgment, appear irritable, excitable, indifferent and so on. Some even lose language expressive ability or the ability to understand language.

P: Oh, that's so terrible! What should I do now?

D: The brain tumor could be malignant or benign, but most of them are benign according to the pathology diagnosis after operation. Surgical treatment is the most basic and effective treatment for intracranial tumors. Radiotherapy, chemotherapy, photodynamic therapy, and thermal therapy are used as appropriate. I recommend that you be admitted to the hospital and accept brain surgery. Surgical treatment includes tumor resection, internal decompression, external decompression, and shortcut surgery. With the development of microsurgery technology, most of the benign intracranial tumors can be completely removed and neurological function can be well protected. Even for malignant tumors, surgical excision alongside other treatments can achieve better results. Palliative operations such as partial resection of tumors, reduction of tumor volume, internal and external decompression, and cerebrospinal fluid shunt can temporarily relieve intracranial hypertension, strive for other treatment opportunities, and prolong the survival time of patients. Is there anything that you wish to ask?

P: Thank you very much. Why do I have a brain tumor? I don't understand! What causes brain tumor?

D: Brain tumor is related to numerous factors. Primarily, it is relevant to genes, such as oncogene and tumor suppressor gene. Activation and overexpression of oncogenes induce tumorigenesis, and the presence and expression of tumor suppressor gene help to inhibit tumorigenesis. Radiation and some chemicals increase the probability of cancer. In addition, viruses can alter genetic characteristics and cause uncontrolled proliferation, leading to cancer.

（2）神经外科重点查体

Assessing the visual system

Acuity: The clinical examination of visual function should begin with the testing of visual acuity. Color vision in each eye should also be tested. Even when visual acuity is normal, patients with lesions of the optic nerve may complain that colors appear "washed out" in the affected eye.

Visual fields: Visual fields in all four quadrants should be tested by comparing the patients' field with the examiner's. Partial or complete visual loss in one eye implies only damage to the retina or optic nerve anterior to the optic chiasm, while a visual field abnormality involving both eyes implies a defect at or posterior to the optic chiasm. A homonymous hemianopia implies a post-chiasmal lesion. Bitemporal hemianopia implies a lesion at the chiasm such as a pituitary tumor. Any suspicious findings on bedside confrontation testing warrant formal visual perimetry testing.

Pupils: Both the direct and indirect light responses should be noted for each eye, such that when the light is shone in one eye both pupils constrict. The accommodative pupillary response is tested by asking the patient to look first in the distance and then at the examiner's finger, held 12 inches away. The pupils should constrict symmetrically and rapidly.

A large unreactive pupil with ptosis indicates a

lesion of the oculomotor nerve (third cranial nerve palsy) interrupting the parasympathetic nerve supply to the pupil. A small unreactive pupil with associated ptosis is known as Hornor's syndrome and results from damage to the sympathetic fibers to the pupil.

Eye movements: Several elements in the history may help in evaluating the patients with diplopia. The examination should begin by determining the position of the head and eyes with the eyes in primary gaze. Disconjugate eye movements suggest a disorder of the brain stem (at the level of the ocular motor nuclei or their connections), peripheral nerves (cranial nerves III, IV, or VI), individual eye muscles (ocular myopathy). The abducens (sixth cranial) nerve supplies the lateral rectus muscle. The trochlear (fourth cranial) nerve sub-serves the superior oblique muscle, which intorts the eye as well as depresses the eye in adduction. All other muscles are supplied by the oculomotor nerve.

（3）重点语句

What kind of headache is it?

How often does it occur?

In which part of the head do you have the headache?

When do the headaches tend to occur?

Do you take a medicine regularly for the headaches?

Do you have an aura, like flickering or blind spot, in the visual field?

Do you experience any abnormal vision?

Do you experience nausea or vomiting?

Does anyone in your family have headaches?

12. 妇 产 科

（1）妇科常见疾病/症状：异常子宫出血 Abnormal Uterine Bleeding

Warming up

Abnormal uterine bleeding(AUB) is a common symptom and sign of gynecology. As a general term, it refers to abnormal bleeding from the uterus that is longer than usual or that occurs at an irregular time. Bleeding may be heavier or lighter than usual and occur often or randomly. It is one of the most common gynecological problems in women of childbearing age. About one third of premenopausal women and more than 70 per cent of all women come to hospital for abnormal uterine bleeding.

The most probable etiology of abnormal uterine bleeding relates to the patient's reproductive age, as does the likelihood of serious endometrial pathology. The specific diagnostic approach depends on whether the patient is premenopausal or postmenopausal. In premenopausal women with normal findings on physical examination, the most likely diagnosis is dysfunctional uterine bleeding (DUB) secondary to anovulation.

If abnormal uterine bleeding is not severe and does not require emergent intervention, evaluation begins with a careful medical history, including the usual menstrual pattern, the extent of recent bleeding, sexual activity, trauma, and symptoms of infection or systemic disease. A complete physical examination, supplemented by laboratory testing, should uncover any signs of systemic disease.

The pelvic examination consists of careful inspection of the lower genital tract for lacerations, vulvar or vaginal pathology, and cervical lesions or polyps. Bimanual uterine examination may reveal enlargement from uterine fibroids, adenomyosis, or endometrial carcinoma.

Laboratory investigation includes pregnancy testing in all patients of reproductive age. A complete blood count provides a measure of blood loss and platelet adequacy. Cervical cultures and a Papanicolaou smear are appropriate initial steps to evaluate for the presence of sexually transmitted diseases or cervical dysplasia.

History taking

Case I

D: Good morning, what can I do for you?

P: *There is something wrong with my period. I think it is 15 days late.*

D: Do you mean you have a delayed period?

P: Yes.

D: When was your last period?

P: Oh, let me see. Probably on March 25th. It is regular most of the time.

D: Was the blood flow the same as usual?

P: It was much less than usual.

D: *What was the color of the bleeding?*

P: It is dark. I would rather call it spotting because the flow was so light.

D: Are you married?

P: Yes, I got married a year ago, and we are trying to have a baby.

D: ***Do you have any other discomforts?***

P: Discomforts? Oh, I do. I feel a little bit painful on the right side of my belly, but not that much.

D: ***How long have you had the pain?***

P: About three days.

D: ***In this case, would you mind if I do a pelvic examination? I think it's necessary.***

P: Sure, no problem.

D: Well, A pelvic exam takes only a few minutes. Take everything off and here is the drape sheet for you to cover your chest. I'll be back when you're ready.

D: (Knock on the door) Are you ready?

P: Yes.

D: Before performing the pelvic exam, I'd like to listen to your heart and lungs.

P: OK.

D: Now, could you lie down on your back and rest your feet on the stirrups?

OK, here is the speculum just like when you have a Pap smear done. You may feel some pressure in your vagina. Just relax as much as possible, but tell me if you're in pain.

P: I see.

D: Well, your uterus is rather soft and a little bit enlarged. Also, I feel that there is a palpable mass in the right abdomen. Now we need a urine sample to see if you got pregnant.

P: Oh, my God, is it possible that I am pregnant? I mean, I am bleeding now.

D: It's possible. Let's have the pregnancy test then we'll start from there.

P: OK.

D: Well, it is weakly positive, which means you are pregnant. Since you have the bleeding and pain in the abdomen, I'd like you to have a transvaginal ultrasound to rule out ectopic pregnancy.

P: Is it severe?

D: ***Don't worry too much now. Let's wait for the ultrasound results.***

P: I will have the ultrasound. I hope there isn't any trouble.

A few minutes later...

D: Well, according to the ultrasound report, the cavity of the uterus is empty, but there is a lump on the right side, and there is some free fluid in the pelvic cavity, which means you may have internal bleeding. To help making the diagnosis accurate, I'm afraid we need to do a further investigation, which is a procedure named culdocentesis.

P: Will that be painful?

D: Maybe slightly. The posterior vaginal fornix is very thin; many patients do not feel any pain during the procedure. Don't worry.

P: OK, I hope it is helpful to find out what is going on.

D: All right, you can see that I've drawn some dark bloody fluid from your abdomen. This bloody fluid does not form clots, which identifies that you have internal bleeding. Based on the symptoms, labs and pelvic exam, it's highly suspected that you have an ectopic pregnancy.

P: Err... how did that happen?

D: Well, there are numerous of risk factors of ectopic

pregnancy. Such as pelvic inflammatory disease, previous ectopic pregnancy, a history of infertility, therapy for in vitro fertilization, increased age, smoking, and using an intra-uterus device. However, a proportion of women with ectopic pregnancy have no identifiable causal factors.

P: OK, what should I do now? Do I need to take any medications?

D: *You should be admitted to the hospital immediately.* Since the mass is already 3 centimeters in diameter, it may rupture at any time. If the rupture occurs, it can be life-threatening. I'll arrange your admission.

P: Oh, I'm lucky that I came to see you. Do I need to have surgery?

D: Based on the results we have now, I think you probably should.

Communication with patient

D: *Having examined you, I am afraid that you have an ectopic pregnancy.*

P: Oh, that's so terrible! What is an ectopic pregnancy?

D: In simple terms, an ectopic pregnancy means "an out-of- place pregnancy". In a normal pregnancy, the fertilized egg moves from the tube into the uterus, where the embryo grows and develops. If this does not happen, the fertilized egg implants and starts to develop outside the uterus, leading to an ectopic pregnancy. An ectopic pregnancy can be life-threatening because as the pregnancy gets bigger it can burst (rupture), causing severe pain and internal bleeding.

You now have abdominal pain, irregular bleeding and other clinical manifestations of ectopic pregnancy.

So, don't worry. I'll admit you to the ward right away in order to start your treatment in time. After a series of workup, you need to have an emergency surgery to stop the bleeding. This operation is often necessary to save the life of the patient. It is done by removing the ruptured fallopian tube and pregnancy. To confirm that you have had an ectopic pregnancy, tissue removed at the time of surgery is sent for testing in the laboratory. As for the type of the surgery for recovery, what you need to do is to relax, don't be worried. Everything will be okay, and we'll take good care of you.

P: OK, I am so nervous and depressed.

D: I fully understand, but don't worry. The doctor who will operate on you is very experienced and considerate. Your doctors will follow-up with you so that they can give you some recommendations and precautions for further pregnancies. If you have any questions, feel free to ask me. You'll be all right.

P: Oh, thank you, doctor. What about my future pregnancies?

D: The chance of having a successful pregnancy in the future is good. Even if you have only one tube, your chance of conceiving is only slightly reduced. For most women an ectopic pregnancy is a 'one-off' event. However, your overall chance of having another ectopic pregnancy is increased and is around $7 \sim 10$ in 100 ($7\% \sim 10\%$) compared with 1 in 90 (just over 1%) in the general Chinese population. It's better that you seek early advice from a healthcare professional when you know you are pregnant. You may need an ultrasound scan between 6 and 8 weeks to confirm that the pregnancy is developing in the uterus. If you do not have a pregnancy desire, seek further advice from your doctor or family planning clinic, as some forms of contraception could be more suitable after an ectopic pregnancy.

Case Ⅱ

D: Good afternoon, I am Dr. Sun. How can I help you?

P: Afternoon Dr. Sun. There is something that scared me. I have abnormal bleeding after I have sex with my husband.

D: Don't worry; I am here trying to help. How old are you?

P: 36.

D: Do you smoke?

P: Yes, I smoke two packs a week.

D: You are married, I see. Do you have any children?

P: Yes, a boy and a girl. The elder is 6 years old and the younger one is 2 years old.

D: Are they healthy?

P: Yes, they are.

D: *Have you been on any medications?*

P: I am currently using birth control pills for contraception. My husband and I have been married for 7 years. We plan to have another baby next year. I am just finishing my menstrual cycle and am spotting. My period is regular without problems.

D: *Have you ever had sexually transmitted diseases?*

P: OK, let me see. I have no history of sexually transmitted diseases.

D: OK. Do you have the bleeding only during intercourse or also under other circumstances (in other situations)?

P: Only during or after I have sex with my husband.

D: And, how many times has it happened?

P: It just started to occur four months ago. It has happened four or five times.

D: *Is the bleeding heavy?*

P: No, it's just some spotting, not too much.

D: *What is the color of the blood?*

P: It's dark.

D: Do you have any other discomforts?

P: No.

D: Do you have abdominal pain?

P: No, I've never had any abdominal pain. But, since you brought up, sometimes I do have some abnormal discharge. It is watery and foul-smelling. I had it several days ago, but now it's gone. I didn't pay attention to it. I have been in good health all my life and seldom go to see a doctor.

D: *Do you get a yearly physical all the time?*

P: Yes, I have received medical care since the age of 17 at the HMC Women's Clinic.

D: OK, I see your establishing care at the HMC Women's Clinic. You are recently engaged and have never had a Pap smear or tests for sexually transmitted diseases or HIV. It's necessary for a woman to have a check-up every year. Sometimes you will not realize that you are ill because some diseases are developing insidiously.

P: I see. What can I do now?

D: Well, I am going to perform a thorough genital and pelvic examination since you have not done one for a long time.

P: OK.

D: Could you please lie down on your back? Just relax and don't be nervous. It might be a little bit of discomfort when I am using a vaginal speculum to expose the cervix.

P: That's fine, doctor.

D: Well, it's done. Your cervix looks relatively normal. Just to be sure, I need to do a Pap smear for further investigation.

P: A Pap smear? How do you do it? Does it hurt?

D: Yes, a Pap smear is part of a pelvic examination. I will scrape a small amount of cells off the surface of your cervix. The cells will be examined under a microscope in a laboratory, where a technician looks at the size and shape of the cells.

P: When can I get the result?

D: ***It takes about 7 days.***

P: Thanks a lot, doctor.

D: You're welcome. Next wednesday, do you prefer 8 o'clock or 10 o'clock?

P: Ten o'clock suits me better

D: If you have time, it will be better to notify us before you come.

P: All right, doctor. I'll see you later. Thank you

D: You are welcome.

Communication with patient

D: Hi, good morning, Mrs. Li.

P: Morning, doctor.

D: I'm sorry to say that things didn't turn out as what we would like they do.

P: Umm...

131

D: Well, your Pap smear result is ready. There is something we need to discuss. The result shows HSIL.

P: What is HSIL?

D: HSIL stands for high-grade squamous intraepithelial lesion. It is an abnormal growth of cells on the cervix. The HSIL can potentially develop to cervical cancer. The diagnosis usually indicates the need for further testing to assess the potential cancer risk.

P: Oh my God.

D: It's not so bad, I can't say exactly what caused this change specifically, I can tell you that several factors can play a role, including smoking, oral contraceptive use, and experience with multiple sexual partners and, of course, having a male partner with multiple sexual partners.

P: I didn't know that.

D: Our standard protocol is to have a colposcopy with endocervical curettage and directed biopsies as indicated. Don't worry too much about it. For most women, an abnormal Pap result is extremely upsetting. However, the diagnosis of a high-grade squamous intraepithelial lesion is found to be cancer in fewer than two percent of cases. It is important to follow-up the diagnosis however, because 20 percent of women with HSIL develop cancer in the future. Aside from the colposcopy and biopsy, more frequent Pap tests are necessary to monitor for changes.

P: Umm...

D: Don't worry, on your way out, please stop at the front desk to arrange your appointment. Of course, if you have any questions after you get home; please feel free to call the clinic. (Looking at the clock on the wall) I'd like to spend more time with you, but we have a very busy schedule this morning.

P: OK, doctor.

（2）妇科重点查体

A pelvic exam usually is done as part of a woman's regular checkup, or your doctor may recommend a pelvic exam if you're having symptoms such as ovarian cysts, sexually transmitted infections, uterine fibroids or early-stage cancer. Doctor checks your vulva, vagina, cervix, uterus, rectum and pelvis, including your ovaries, for masses, growths or other abnormalities. A Pap test, which screens for cervical cancer, may be performed during a pelvic exam.

Speculum exam

Vulva: looking for irritation, redness, sores, swelling, or any other abnormalities.

External genitalia: looking for irritation, redness, sores, swelling, or any other abnormalities. Normal appearance is no enlargement of the Bartholin or Skene glands.

Urethra and bladder are non-tender.

Vagina: discharge, order, color, lesion. The normal is clean, without lesions or discharge.

Cervix: color, shape, position. The normal is smooth, without lesions.

Palpate

Cervix：position, shape, consistency, regularity, mobility and tenderness. Motion of the cervix causes no pain.

Uterus: size, position, consistency, mobility, tenderness, normal uterus is the size of a small orange. When enlarged often described in size corresponding to weeks of pregnancy, firm, smooth surface, anteverted (80%) and anteflexed. Freely movable. Not tender.

Adnexa (tubes and ovaries): size, consistency, mobility, tenderness, and enlarge. **Normal:** Ovary 2cm× 2cm, almond shaped, slightly tender to palpation, very mobile, tubes and ovaries are neither tender nor enlarged.

（3）产科常见疾病/症状：产前出血 Antepartum Hemorrhage

Warming up

Antepartum hemorrhage (APH) complicates 2%～ 5% of pregnancies and is defined in some literature as any bleeding from the genital tract after the 28th week of pregnancy and before labor. It is three times as common in multifarious women as in primiparae. The incidence increases with each previous caesarean section. An APH may also be retained in the uterus. Identifiable causes of APH are recognized in 50% of cases, and in the other 50% of cases the cause for the APH is indeterminate or unknown. It commonly arises from the placenta as placenta praevia, placental abruption, or it can come from a vasa praevia or local lesions in the cervix or vagina but this is very rare. It is not uncommon to fail to identify a cause for APH when it is then described as "unexplained APH". It is crucial to distinguish between these causes from the outset as their definitive management could differ significantly. Early diagnosis is also extremely important to ensure prompt institution of management.

Blood loss if often underestimated and the amount visible may only be a portion of the total volume of the hemorrhage (e.g. with a concealed placental abruption), therefore clinicians immediately need to assess not only the amount of blood loss, but also observe for signs of maternal clinical shock and fetal compromise or demise. Women with a history of APH are at increased risk for adverse prenatal outcomes including small for gestational age and growth restricted fetuses, therefore initiation of serial ultrasounds is recommended. Other risk factors include increased risk for oligohydramnios, premature rupture of membranes, preterm labor and increased rates of caesarean section. Women diagnosed with placental abruption or placental praevia are at increased risk for postpartum hemorrhage. APH from unknown causes before 34 weeks gestation is associated with a 60% chance of birth within a week if accompanied by contractions. Without accompanying contractions, the chance is still 13.6%, therefore administration of corticosteroids is important.

History taking

Case I

D: Hi, how can I help you, Mrs. Jones?

P: Hello, Doctor. I am 35 weeks pregnant with my second child. I'm worried. I'm not feeling well today.

D: Relax and don't worry. What's your concerns?

P: There's a little vaginal bleeding and abdominal pain today.

D: ***Try to relax, when was your last menstrual period?***

P: Oh, let me see. I think it was on Apr 2nd, and on time.

D: *Do you have regular menstrual cycles?*

P: Yes, I have a regular cycle all the time.

D: OK, I see. So, your gestational age is 34 weeks, and the due date is 09/01/2019, right?

P: Yes, but I have bloody discharge from this morning.

D: Can you describe the discharge? Is it less than, equal to, or greater than your normal period? What's changed? Did it start suddenly?

P: It's slight, spotting, like the first few hours when I have my period. I felt horrible, coupled with a pain in my belly.

D: How long have you had the bleeding and pain?

P: It started in the morning. At the beginning, I had a backache with vaginal spotting.

D: How long has the backache lasted?

P: About 3 hours, but this afternoon it moved to the lower part of the abdomen. It has been 5 hours since then.

D: *Have you ever had this pain before? What is the severity of the pain (sharp, dull, tender, cramping, burning)? Is it intermittent or continuous? Does the pain travel anywhere (radiate) or is it localized?*

P: Honestly it felt like a really tight sensation in my abdomen. My stomach would get as hard as a rock, and when this happened, I lost my breath, I couldn't talk, and I could barely move. However, this wasn't severely painful, just a little cramping. At first, they were continuous (about every 25 minutes). I am so worried about my baby. Is it still okay? Is the baby coming out soon?

D: Relax and take a deep breath. Have you ever had

any watery discharge?

P: No, just spotting.

D: Have you had any other symptoms? Like back pain or pressure?

P: I don't know. I did have a backache; but it was mild so I didn't pay attention to that. It was two days ago.

D: *How was your last pregnancy?*

P: My first child was 3 years old and born at 37 weeks but was 3 500g (full term according to the doctor but still made me worrisome) and I was diagnosed with bacterial vaginosis early on in that pregnancy. My water broke but I didn't start laboring and had to be induced with IV Pitocin. I'm pregnant the second time and I'm wondering if this one will be early as well. It's always nerve-racking when thinking that there's a possibility something could happen to my child.

D: *How about the fetal movement? Is it like normal?*

P: Everything has been going normal with this pregnancy. I felt the baby quickening around 17 weeks and since then it has steadily increased to the point of painful kicks and punches and sometimes rolls.

D: Let me administer a non-stress test for you. The test is usually done to see the baby's well-being and the contraction of uterus. It will take at least 20 minutes in an exam room. OK, please sit in the chair with fetal monitoring equipment hooked to your belly. The monitor will record your baby's heart rate in conjunction with any uterine activity. Click the button when the baby moves so that the heart rate can be seen in relation to that movement.

P: OK, doctor, I'm so nervous.

D: *Try to relax, do you have regular prenatal care with our hospital?*

P: Yes, and everything is OK.

D: OK, I've received your prenatal care record already. You don't have placenta praevia according to the ultrasound report. Don't worry about the baby. The fetal heart is beating strongly and regularly, while the contractions are getting stronger and more regularly. You have contractions every 2 to 3 minutes, even though you don't realize it. You should time from the start of one contraction to the start of the next contraction, it indicates how far apart your contractions are coming. Generally, the early contractions are pre-labor kind of stuff, and may last 20 to 30 seconds at most. But when the contraction lasts close to a minute, and the interval becomes consistently about four minutes apart, and this condition has been going on for an hour, that's when you're in labor. So, I think that you may go into a preterm labor. Let me check your cervix for dilation. You may feel some discomfort.

P: Mm-hmm, all right.

D: The cervix is dilated 3 centimeters. Dilation is the opening up of the cervix and is measured in centimeters. A fingertip dilated means about 1 centimeter dilated. Full dilation is 10 centimeters. Once full dilation occurs, the cervix is completely gone and over the baby's head; and you may push the baby out to be born. Oh, I can feel the amniotic sac, aka the bag of the water through the vagina. It is intact so you didn't have the watery discharge. Given that you may be going into preterm labor soon. I need to admit you to the hospital right now.

P: Oh, my God, I am only 35weeks pregnant! What about the baby?

D: Don't worry about your baby. You will be admitted to the delivery room soon. Your baby will be evaluated carefully and we'll take a good care of him.

Communication with patient

D: According to all the examinations and tests results, I'm afraid that you're having a preterm labor.

P: What is a preterm labor? What does that mean for me and my baby?

D: If labor occurs before 37 weeks of pregnancy, it's defined as preterm labor. In order to have true premature labor, two things need to happen: you must have contractions as well as changes in the cervix, such as thinning out or dilation and you must have regular contraction and cervix dilated, so you are in preterm labor.

Early labor usually happens spontaneously, but it can also be induced for medical reasons, such as if the mother has preeclampsia, a combination of high blood pressure and a kidney and liver problem in the mother. Preterm labor puts baby at risk for a premature birth, which, in turn, increases the chance that the infant will have health complications such as a low birth weight, breathing difficulties, under developed organs, an increased risk of vision or hearing problems, a higher chance of behavioral disabilities and learning problems.

In generally, the more mature a baby is at birth, the better the chance of surviving and being healthy. Something else that's reassuring is that not all premature babies go on to have complications. A baby who is born closer to the 37-week mark has a greater chance of being healthy. But you do see signs of preterm labor and it does look like you'll deliver prior to 35 weeks. You should be given corticosteroid injections, which helps speed up the development of baby's lungs, decreases the chance of dangerous breathing complications, and other problems associated with immature lungs. You should also be given magnesium sulfate, which can help reduce the risk of cerebral palsy in preterm infants.

P: Can it be stopped?

D: There's no surefire way to stop it once it's started. However, you should be admitted to our hospital and rest in bed as much as possible. You should be monitored for the baby's heartbeat and given Ⅳ fluids a medication called a tocolytic, which relaxes the uterine smooth muscle to help slow down or temporarily halt contractions. The contractions and labor could stop completely; I will keep you in the hospital for a while longer to ensure that the cervix isn't continuing to dilate before sending you home.

If you have any question please don't hesitate to ask me. We are here to do everything we can to help you and your baby.

P: Thanks a lot, doctor.

Case Ⅱ

D: Hello, I am Dr. Wang, I am on duty for taking care of you today. How can I help you?

P: Hi Dr. Wang, I am 31 weeks pregnant, and was hit by a motorcycle half an hour ago.

D: Oh, I am sorry to hear that. Can I start by asking you some questions?

P: Sure.

D: Do you have any abdominal pain? Do you have any vaginal bleeding?

P: I felt a little bit of tightness of my belly, without bleeding at the first few minutes. But after a while, I would say maybe 5 minutes later, I started to have some vaginal bleeding, but the amount was very small.

D: How would you describe the pain? Was it dull or sharp? Was it intermittent or constant? Can you point to me where the pain is at?

P: Yes, it right here. At first, the pain was slight, and later on, it became stronger and stronger. It was not constant but the interval became shorter and shorter. It happens almost every 4~5 minutes currently.

D: I see. Is this your first pregnancy?

P: Yes, this is the first time for me to be pregnant.

D: ***Do you have regular prenatal care?***

P: Sure, I have my prenatal care with this hospital. I always follow my physician's instructions. Everything had been fine until I had this accident.

D: Can you describe what happened during the accident in detail?

P: OK, about half hour ago, when I was walking across the intersection, a motorcyclist was speeding and hit the right side of my body. I was knocked over, with my belly touching the ground first.

D: ***Did you feel dizzy or have a headache after the incident (at that time)?***

P: No, I thought I was fine in the first few minutes. But I felt a little bit tight when my baby moved more often than usual. So I called 120 to send me here to find out if there is anything wrong with my baby and me. I am still nervous.

D: Don't worry, what you need to do now is to relax. It is helpful to you and your baby.

P: Thank you, doctor.

D: *How about the fetal movement? Is it more frequent?*

P: Yeah, it kicked me harder and moved more frequently.

D: Would you mind if I take a look and do a physical examination so that I can get more information?

P: Sure.

D: Please lie down on your back. Your abdomen is a little bit tight and I can feel the movement of the baby. I think I need to have you to do some tests to evaluate the status of the baby, and to evaluate the chance of a preterm labor. It will take at least 20 minutes. In addition, I think it is necessary to have an ultrasound and blood tests to rule out placental abruption.

Communication with patient

D: OK, we've got all the results. I'm afraid that you're suspected to have a placental abruption. Patients with suspected placental abruption should be admitted for workup until deemed clinically stable and ready for discharge or outpatient follow-up, or they should stay in hospital and may deliver for medical indications.

P: What is placental abruption? What does that mean for me and my baby?

D: The placenta connects the growing baby to the mother's uterus. It acts as a "lifeline" that gives food and oxygen to the baby through the umbilical cord. Placental abruption happens when the placenta separates from the uterus before the baby is born, with blood collecting between the placenta and the uterus. In most cases, the placenta stays attached to the uterus. In the case of placental abruption, this lifeline is placed at risk.

Placental abruption can be life-threatening to your baby and sometimes to you as well. It can lead to premature birth, low birth weight, blood loss in the mother, and in rare cases, it can cause the baby's death. About 1 out of 100 pregnancies has placental abruption. This condition is usually seen in the third trimester, but it can also happen after 20 weeks of pregnancy. It is one of the two most common causes of antepartum hemorrhage (the other being placenta praevia) which account for 30% of all cases of antepartum hemorrhage.

P: Oh, that sounds so terrible! I am only 31weeks! What about my baby?

D: I think you should be admitted to the hospital immediately. I'm going to make arrangements for your admission. Your doctor will consult with pediatric clinicians, notify NICU, and prepare resuscitation equipment appropriate for gestational age.

P: What should I do right now? Do I need take any medications?

D: As a general rule, once the placenta has separated from the uterus, it cannot be repaired. The treatment depends on the amount of bleeding, how long the pregnancy is, how old the baby is, and the pain in you. After admission, your doctor will monitor you and your baby's vital signs. However, severe cases or unstable patients may require intense care unit admission with readiness for surgical interventions, especially if undelivered. If an emergency happens, the baby will be delivered by Caesarean section.

P: Oh, thank you, doctor.

（4）产科重点查体

Abdominal Examination

1) Inspection

The apparent size of the abdominal distension, edema, or calf tenderness (any asymmetry).

Linea nigra (dark pigmented line stretching from the Xiphi sternum through the umbilicus to the suprapubic area).

Striae gravidarum (recent stretch marks are purplish in color).

Striae albicans (old stretch marks are silvery-white).

Flattening/eversion of umbilicus (due to intra-abdominal pressure).

Superficial veins.

Surgical scars, previous caesarean section, laparoscopic port scars.

2) Palpation

Symphysis-fundal height (SFH): palpated < 20 weeks, measured in cm > 20 weeks.

Number of fetuses

Fetal lie (relationship of longitudinal axis of fetus to that of the uterus): Longitudinal-fetal head or breech palpable over pelvic inlet. Oblique-the head or breech is palpable in the iliac fossa. Transverse-fetal poles felt in flanks. Presentation (part of the fetus overlying the pelvic brim): cephalic, breech, other (shoulder, compound).

Uterus contraction: ①Assessment of contraction patterns is qualitative and can be performed with an external tocodynamometer or tocotransducer (Toco), whereas quantitative measurement of uterine strength requires an internal uterine pressure catheter (IUPC). ②Qualitative patterns include regular uterine contractions, Braxton Hicks contractions, tachysystole, paired contractions, skewed contractions, tetanic contractions, and uterine hypertonus. ③In most normal spontaneous labors, contractions occur with a frequency of 2~5 minutes, and they may last between 30~60 seconds. The ascent and descent of the contraction are gradual and similar to one another. Contractions tend to become stronger and more frequent as labor progresses. Such a contraction pattern would be denoted as regular uterine contractions, with a commentary on the frequency of the contractions (e.g., every 2~3 minutes).

3）Auscultation of the fetal heart: 110~160 beats per minites

Fetal heart rate monitoring: uterine contractions, baseline fetal heart rate, baseline heart rate, baseline variability, presences accelerations, periodic or episodic decelerations. Periodic: associated with contractions; Episodic: not associated with contractions, changes/ trend in the fetal heart rate pattern over time.

Engagement (maximum diameter pass through pelvic inlet): yes or no.

Vaginal examination: (or speculum) is not part of a routine obstetric examination but may be indicated to diagnose rupture of membranes or onset of labor.

Edema or calf tenderness.

（5）重点语句

Abnormal Uterine Bleeding

There is something wrong with my period. I think it is 15 days late.

What is the color of the bleeding?

Do you have any other discomforts? Like abdominal pain?

How long have you been like this?

In that case, would you mind if I do a pelvic examination? I think it's necessary.

Don't worry too much now. Let's wait for the ultrasound results.

You need to be admitted to the hospital immediately.

Having examined you, I am afraid that you have an ectopic pregnancy.

Have you been on any medications?

Would you please tell me about your past illnesses?

Is the bleeding heavy? What is the color of the blood?

Do you get a yearly physical all the time?

It takes about 7 days.

I'm sorry to say that things didn't turn out as we would have liked.

Antepartum Hemorrhage

Relax and don't worry. Where don't you feel well?

When was your last menstrual period? Do you have regular menstrual cycles?

What is the severity of the pain (sharp, dull, tender, cramping, burning)? Is it intermittent or constant?

Does the pain travel anywhere (radiate) or is it localized?

Do you have regular prenatal care with our hospital?

How was your last pregnancy?

How about your fetal movement?

Did you feel dizzy or have a headache after the incident (at that time)?

Have you ever had an abortion before? Do you have regular prenatal care?

13. 儿　　科

（1）儿科常见症状 / 疾病：发热 Fever

Warming up

Fever, one of the most important and common presenting manifestations in children, occurs in response to the release of endogenous pyogenic mediators which are called cytokines. Fever plays a critical role in fighting infections. Although it may be uncomfortable, fever does not necessitate treatment in an otherwise healthy child.

The causes of fever remarkably differ based on whether the fever is acute ($\leq$ 14 days), acute recurrent or periodic (episodes of fever are separated by afebrile periods), or chronic (>14 days). A chronic fever is more commonly referred to as "fever of unknown origin".

The response to antipyretics and the temperature have no direct relationship to the etiology or its seriousness. The significance of fever depends on the clinical context rather than the peak temperature;

some minor diseases may cause a high fever, whereas some serious diseases may just cause mild temperature elevations.

The following factors are of particular concern:

ⅰ) Age < 1 month

ⅱ) Lethargy, listlessness, or toxic appearance

ⅲ) Respiratory distress

ⅳ) Petechiae or purpura

ⅴ) Inconsolability

History taking

D: Hello, Mrs. Liu, how may I help you?

P: My daughter has a fever.

D: What is her name?

P: Her name is xxx.

D: ***How old is she?***

P: She is 18 months old.

D: ***When did she get the fever?***

P: It started two days ago.

D: Have you taken her temperature?

P: Yes, I have. It was 38.3 ℃ by a forehead thermometer.

D: ***Is the fever constant or on and off?***

P: I think that she has a constant fever. Tylenol works well on her, but only for a couple of hours, then her temperature goes up above 38 ℃ again.

D: I am sorry to hear that. Does she have a runny nose?

P: Not currently, but she did have a runny nose for a few days about a week ago.

D: ***Has she pulled at her ears***?

P: Yes, she has been pulling at her right ear for two

days.

D: Has there been any discharge from her ears?

P: No.

D: Does she have a cough?

P: Not currently, but she was coughing for a few days about a week ago.

D: *Has she had shortness of breath?*

P: No.

D: Has she had difficulty swallowing?

P: She seems to have trouble swallowing, but I am not sure.

D: *Does she have a rash on her body*?

P: Yes, she has a rash on her face and chest.

D: Could you describe her rash in detail, please?

P: Tinny red dots, some slightly elevated, over the chest, back, belly, and face. There is no rash on her arms or legs.

D: *When did her rash start?*

P: It started two days ago.

D: *Have you noticed on which part of the body the rash started?*

P: It started on her face and then spread to her chest, back and belly.

D: Does she have nausea and vomiting?

P: Yes, she vomited last night.

D: Does she have any changes in bowel habits, in stool color, or consistency?

P: No.

D: Has she had any changes in urinary habits or in urine smell or color?

P: No.

D: *Has she had chills or seizures?*

P: No.

D: *Has she been lethargic, irritated, active, etc.?*

P: She looks tired. She doesn't plays with her toys or watches TV the way she usually does.

D: Has her appetite changed?

P: She does not eat much but is able to drink milk.

D: *Has she come into contact with anyone sick?*

P: No.

D: *What about her vaccinations?*

P: Up to date.

D: When was her last checkup?

P: One month ago, and everything was normal.

D: Could you tell me if there were any problems at her delivery, please?

P: It was a 40-week vaginal delivery without any problems.

D: How is her weight, height, and language development?

P: Normal.

D: Could you tell me about her diet, please?

P: Whole milk and solid food; I didn't do breastfeeding.

D: How about her sleep patterns?

P: She has not slept well for 2 days.

D: Has she had hearing problems?

P: No.

D: Has she had vision problems?

P: No.

D: Is she taking any medications currently?

P: Her current medication is just Tylenol.

D: Does she have any past medical histories?

P: Three months ago, she had an ear infection which was treated successfully with amoxicillin.

D: Has she had any surgeries in the past?

P: No.

D: Does she have any drug allergies?

P: No.

Communication and interpretations

D: Mrs. Liu. It appears that your daughter is suffering from an infection or something more serious which can be caused by viruses or bacteria.

P: Could you please tell me more about her condition?

D: Yes. She may have an acute upper respiratory infection (URI) and an acute otitis media, because she has fever, pulling at her right ear, fatigue, and past history with ear infection. Children with URI are prone to secondary otitis media. However, some other differential diagnoses should be excluded, such as meningococcal meningitis and scarlet fever. Therefore, a physical exam and some preliminary blood tests are needed, including CBC with differential and C reaction protein. If her fever persists, further auxiliary examinations will be done to identify the source of infection and the type of viruses or bacteria involved, such as chest X-ray, throat culture, pneumatic otoscopy, platelets, PT/APTT, D-dimer, fibrin split products, fibrinogen, blood culture, and cerebrospineal fluid analysis.

P: What treatment will you give her?

D: Although viral infections generally clear on its own, most bacterial infections require antibiotics. Such infections generally respond well to treatment. I will decide whether to apply antibiotics based on her test results. Do you have any more questions for me?

P: No. I got it. Thank you very much.

（2）儿科常见症状 / 疾病: 咳嗽 Cough

Warming up

A cough is a reflex that helps clear the airways of secretions, protects the airway from foreign body aspiration. A cough is one of the most common complaints for which parents bring their children to see doctor.

Causes of a cough vary depending on whether the symptoms are acute (< 2 weeks) or chronic (> 4 weeks). For an acute cough, the most common cause is viral upper respiratory infection (URI). For a chronic cough, the most common causes include cough variant asthma (CVA, the most common), post-infectious cough (PIC), upper airway cough syndrome (UACS), gastroesophageal reflux disorder (GERD), and psychogenic cough. Foreign body aspiration and diseases such as non-asthma eosinophilic bronchitis and atopic cough are less common, although they can all result in persistent cough.

The following factors are of particular concern:

ⅰ) Cyanosis or hypoxia on pulse oximetry

ⅱ) Stridor

ⅲ) Respiratory distress

ⅳ) Toxic appearance

ⅴ) Abnormal lung examination

History taking

D: Hello, sit down please, Mrs. Wang. What's troubling your son?

P: He has a cough and a fever.

D: What's his name?

P: His name is XX.

D: How old is he?

P: He is 2 years old.

D: ***When did it start?***

P: It started 4 days ago with a runny nose. The fever and cough started 3 days ago.

D: ***Is it constant or intermittent?***

P: It is constant.

D: ***How often does he cough?***

P: He has been coughing and with a fever the whole time.

D: How severe is the fever?

P: I just measured 39.8℃.

D: By what means?

P: I did it with the ear thermometer.

D: Has he had any chills or seizures?

P: No.

D: ***Does anything make it better or worse?***

P: I gave him Tylenol. It lowered his temperature.

D: ***Does anything come up when he coughs?***

P: None.

D: ***Is the cough or fever getting better, getting worse, or staying the same?***

P: The fever has gotten worse, and he has been coughing more since it started.

D: ***Have you noticed if his skin pulls in or out between each rib or below the ribs with each breath?***

P: No.

D: ***Has he had shortness of breath?***

P: He is breathing faster than usual.

D: *Has he had noisy breathing?*

P: No.

D: *Has he turned blue around his lips or mouth?*

P: No.

D: Has he ever had this cough before?

P: He gets sick pretty often. The last time he had a cough was about 3 months ago. But he didn't have such a high fever then.

D: Has he had any other symptoms, such as rash, ear/eye discharge, ear pulling, difficulty swallowing or speaking?

P: He also has diarrhea. I haven't seen any rashes. He hasn't had any discharge, ear pulling, or difficulty swallowing or speaking.

D: When did his diarrhea start?

P: It started 2 days ago.

D: How often?

P: He has 4~5 poopy diapers per day.

D: What is the color of the stools?

P: Normal color.

D: Any blood in stools?

P: No.

D: Are the stools poorly formed?

P: They're watery.

D: Has he had nausea or vomiting?

P: No.

D: Has he had any problems with urination?

P: No.

D: Has he had sleep problems?

P: He hasn't been sleeping well, because he is really

uncomfortable.

D: How about his activity?

P: He is really not his normal self at all. Usually, he is active.

D: Has he been lethargic or sleepy?

P: No, nothing like that. He just seems really upset.

D: Has he had dry mouth or sunken eyes?

P: It seems like he has a dry mouth, and he's been drinking less than normal.

D: ***Has he travelled recently?***

P: No.

D: Could you tell me his past medical history?

P: He had jaundice for the first week after he was born. He was treated with blue light.

D: Has he ever had any surgeries in the past?

P: None.

D: Does he have any allergies?

P: None.

D: How did the pregnancy go?

P: Normal.

D: Has he been taking any medications?

P: No.

D: Has he come in contact with anyone sick?

P: He's been staying at home with me. His older brother goes to kindergarten and has been sick for 4 days. He has a runny nose and cough too, but no fever.

D: Were there any problems at the delivery?

P: He was born vaginally at 37 weeks. There were no problems whatsoever.

D: How about his immunizations?

P: All of his immunizations are up-to-date.

D: How about his growth and development?

P: Everything has been normal so far.

D: Has his eating habits or appetite changed?

P: He usually eats everything I give him, including meat, vegetables, fruits, and bread. But he hasn't been eating well the past few days.

D: What about his last checkup?

P: He had a checkup one month ago and everything was fine.

Communication and interpretation

D: Mrs. Wang. I understand how you are feeling. According to what you have told me, I think that your son may have a serious infection that requires treatment.

P: What could it be?

D: Based on his presentations, I think that he probably has an acute bronchitis. This is the most likely cause of his cough and fever. Acute bronchitis is oftentimes preceded by an upper respiratory infection (URI), which is what your son had. Acute bronchitis is caused by viral infection in > 90% of cases and as such does not usually require antibiotic treatment. Adenovirus is known for causing both respiratory, stomach, and bowel symptoms, which are consistent with your son's condition. However, we need to do some tests to rule out pneumonia and viral gastroenteritis, as well as influenza and sepsis.

P: What tests does he need?

D: First, I will do physical examinations on him, then I will suggest some blood tests, including CBC with differential, respiratory viral panel, arterial blood gas analysis, electrolytes, glucose, and a chest X ray, Do you have more questions, Mrs. Wang?

P: No, thank you.

（3）儿科重点查体

1) Vitals: Temperature (tympanic, oral, axillary, rectal), heart rate or pulse, respiration rate, O_2 saturation, blood pressure, growth parameters (weight, height, growth curve, body mass index).

2) General: Nutritional status, level of consciousness, toxic or distressed, cyanosis, cooperation, hydration, dysmorphology, mental state.

3) Skin and Lymphatics: Color, jaundice, rashes, petechiae, desquamation, pigmentation, texture, turgor, lymph node enlargement, location, mobility, consistency.

4) Head and Neck

Nose, eye, and/or ear discharge; vision; hearing.

Mouth and throat: Lips color, buccal mucosa (color, vesicles, moist or dry), tongue (color, papillae, position, tremors), teeth and gums (number, condition), palate (intact, arch), tonsils (size, color, exudates), posterior pharyngeal wall (color, lymph hyperplasia, bulging), gag reflex, herpes of the mouth.

Neck: Thyroid, trachea position, masses (cysts, nodes), presence or absence of nuchal rigidity.

5) Lungs/Thorax

Inspection: Pattern of breathing, respiratory rate, use of accessory muscles (retraction location, degree/flaring), chest wall configuration.

Auscultation: Equality of breath sounds; rales, wheezes, rhonchi, upper airway noise.

Percussion and palpation: Often not possible or rarely helpful.

6) Cardiovascular

Auscultation: Rhythm, murmurs, quality of heart sounds.

Pulses: Quality in upper and lower extremities.

7) Abdomen

Inspection: Shape, umbilicus (infection, hernias), muscular integrity (diastasis recti).

Auscultation: Bowel sounds.

Palpation: Tenderness, avoid the tender area until the end of exam, liver, spleen, kidneys, rebound, guarding.

8) Musculoskeletal

Back: Sacral dimple, kyphosis, lordosis or scoliosis.

Joints: motion, stability, swelling, tenderness.

Extremities: Deformity, symmetry, edema, clubbing.

Gait: In-toeing, out-toeing, bowed legs, knocking knees, limp.

Hips: Ortolani's and Barlow's signs.

9) Neurologic-most accomplished through observation alone

Cranial nerves

Sensation

Cerebellar/ coordination

Muscle tone and strength

Reflexes: deep tendon reflex, superficial (abdominal and cremasteric), neonatal primitive.

Babinski sign, Oppenheim sign, Kerning sign, Brudzinski sign.

（4）重点语句

Fever

How old is she?

When did her fever begin?

Is her fever constant or on and off?

Has she pulled at her ears?

Has she had shortness of breath?

Does she have rash on her body?

When did her rash start?

Did you notice on which part of her body the rash started?

Does she have seizures?

How does she look? Lethargic, irritated, active, etc.?

Did she come into contact with anyone sick?

What about her vaccinations?

Cough

When did it start?

Is it constant or intermittent?

How often does he cough?

Does anything make it better or worse?

Does anything come up when he coughs?

Is the cough or fever getting better, getting worse, or staying the same?

Do you notice if his skin pulls in or out between each rib or below the ribs with each breath?

Has he had shortness of breath?

Has he had noisy breathing?

Has he turned blue around his lips or mouth?

Has he travelled recently?

第三章 病历书写及病例报告写作
Chapter 3. Medical Record and Case Report Writing

1. 病历内容 Contents of Medical Records

（1）基本信息 General Data: Such as name, sex, age, native, birth place, profession, marital status, source of history and estimate of reliability etc.

（2）主诉 Chief Complaints: It should constituted by a few simple words why the patient consulted his physician, which usually includes symptoms or sign the patient is suffering and the duration time.

（3）现病史 Present Illness: It should be a well-organized, sequentially developed elaboration of patient's chief complaints. A good medical history will reflect the diagnosis or impression which is going to be made.

It includes the following aspects:

1) Onset and duration of the disease.

2) Main symptoms, location and their characters.

3) Both provoking and releasing factors.

4) Evolution of disease.

5) Associated symptoms.

6) Medical treatment and its effects.

7) General condition, especially the dietary habit.

（4）既往史 Past History: Health condition and disease which the patient suffered before the present illness. Infectious disease, surgery, allergy are essential part of the past history.

（5）系统回顾 Systems Review

The purpose of this review is twofold:

1) A thorough evaluation of the past and present status of every system.

2) A double check to prevent omission of significant data relative to the present illness.

（6）个人史 Personal History: It includes those information that relating to smoking and alcoholic beverages (duration and amount), sedatives, social history, profession and working condition.

（7）婚姻史 Marital History: This review includes data concerning the health of the mate, the number of children and their physical status.

（8）月经史和生育史 Menstrual History and Childbearing history: It applies to women only. It should include the menarche age and the condition of giving birth.

（9）家族史 Family History: Inquire the disease of patient's first relative which might be hereditary, such as heart disease, hypertension, diabetes etc.

2. 英文病历常用表述方式 Terminologies in Medical Records

（1）症状发作

complain of

have a feeling (sensation) of...

suffer from

have an attack of

have (fell)

begin to fell

（2）疾病诱因

- 无诱因　with no inducing factors
- 无明显诱因 under no obvious predisposing causes
- 感冒一周后 after getting (catching) common cold for 1 week
- 活动时呼吸困难 dyspnea on exertion
- 与……有关 be associated with have (make) relation to
- 与……无关 have (make) no relation to
- 伴发　be accompanied by

（3）起病方式

- 突发胸痛 an explosive onset of chest pain
- 急性腹痛 acute abdominal pain
- 持续性胸痛 chest pain continually
- 反复胸闷心悸 recurrent (bouts of) chest discomfort and palpitation
- 频发胸痛 frequent episodes of chest pain
- 发作性呼吸困难 paroxysmal short of breath
- 慢性低热 chronic lower fever
- 突然起病伴高热 the onset was sudden with high fever
- 因……而突然发作 the attack is precipitated by...
- 很快发生 occured rapidly
- 偶尔 occasionally , sporadically, accidentally
- 逐渐出现咳嗽咳痰 gradual onset of cough and sputum
- 一过性发作 transitory attack

- 频繁 frequently
- 持续性（间歇性）persistent (intermittent)

（4）病情变化描述

- 好转
  fell better than before
  be better
  take a favorable turn
  improve
  turn for the better
- 症状减轻
  alleviate
  reduce
  palliate
  diminish
- 症状消失
  relieve
  disappear
  regress
  clear up
  vanish
  dissolve
- 症状加重
  be (become, get) worse
  worsen
  take a turn for the worse
  be aggravated
  increase in severity
  take a bad turn
- 无变化
  be alike

be similar

continue without change

be identical

resemble

- 体温／血压升降

升至 rise (go up) to

已升至 have risen (gone up) to

升至 be elevated to

已降至 have gone down (dropped) to

骤降（升）sudden drop (elevation)

渐降（升）fall (elevate) gradually

降至正常 drop (was reduced) to normal

恢复到正常 return (revert) to normal

维持在……水平 maintain at a level of...

稳定在…… stabilize at...

不超过 do not go up over (exceed)...

在……和……之间波动 fluctuate (vary) between...and...

（5）时间

- 持续

lasted for 3 days

lasted on the average 3～5 minutes

have continued for 10 hours

lasted about half an hour

- 超过（不到）move than (less than)
- 多在……时发生 usually in the morning
- 未发作过 be free of onsets (attacks) for 2 weeks

（6）严重程度

- 轻度 mild (slight)

- 中度 moderate
- 重度 severe (serious)

（7）其他描述方法

- 部位
  位于 be located (situated) in (over)
  疼痛位于 There is localized pain in...
  在……附近 near...
  局限于 be localized to (in, over)
  局限于 be limited (confined) to
- 表示部位的介词
  心尖部，表示小的部位或点 at the apex
  上腹部，表示大的部位 in the upper abdomen
  在左下肢，表示皮肤表面上（下）的病变 on (beneath) the left lower limb
  在右肺，表示正上方的相应体表部位 over the right lung
  嘴上（下）方，表示高低或上下的位置关系 above (below) the mouth
  左乳皮下 under the skin of the left breast
- 转移 / 放射
  转移到…… shift (migrate) to...
  放射到…… radiate (travel, go, refer)to...
  从……放射到…… radiate from...to...
- 耳鼻咽喉及口腔症状
  耳痛 otalgia (pain of ears)
  耳鸣 tinnitus (ears ring)
  耳鸣 the perception of noise in the ear or head
  耳聋 deafness (loss in hearing)
  耳流脓 otorrhea (otopyorrhea)

耳出血 otorrhagia

耳垢 cerumen (earwax)

耳血肿 othematoma

鼻塞 nasal obstruction

不能用鼻呼吸 unable to breathe through (by) the nose (nasal dyspnea)

打喷嚏和流涕 sneezing and nasal discharge

水样鼻涕 watery rhinorrhea

鼻出血 nosebleed

咽喉痛 sore throat

口吃 stuttering

口臭 ozostomia (saburra, halitosis)

吞咽困难 difficult in swallowing

咽下困难 dysphagia

流涎多 have excessive salvation

- 眼科及牙科症状

眼睑水肿 eyelid edema

眼痛 pain in the eye

过度流泪 excessive tearing (watering)

视疲劳 asthenopia (visional tired)

视力减退 hypopsia (diminution of vision)

视力衰弱 ophthalmocopia

远（近）视力模糊 indistinct distant (near) vision

失明 loss of vision

搏动性牙痛 throbbing pain of tooth (odontalgia)

牙龈出血 gingival bleeding

牙龈萎缩（增生）gingival atrophy(hypertrophy)

- 妇产科症状

经量少（中等、多）mild (moderate, heavy) menses

月经过少 hypomenorrhea

阴道出血 vaginal bleeding(colporrhagia)

月经规则（不规则）regular (irregular) menstrual cycle

月经周期 26 天，持续 4 天 menstrual periods of 26 days and lasted 4 days

白带增多 leukorrhagia (profuse leukorrhea or whites)

绝经 amenorrhea

停经 menopause

经前（期）痛 menstruation cramp

预产期 expected date of labor

羊水过多（少）polyhydramnios (oligohydramnios)

月经期水肿 menstrual edema

月经失调 menstrual disorder

性欲正常（减退）normal (decreased) libido

产程 stage of labor

产程延长 prolonged labor

产前出血 antepartum hemorrhage

产前子痫 prenatal eclampsia

产前检查 prenatal examination

妊娠呕吐 vomiting of pregnancy (hyperemesis gravidarum)

妊娠反应 pregnancy reaction

妊娠高血压（水肿）gestation hypertension (edema)

- 病程中的一般情况

一般情况尚可（一般、差）general condition is fair (ordinary, bad)

胃纳佳（差）have a good (poor) appetite

多食 eat too much (overeat, eat heavily)

少食 eat poorly (take little food)

167

食欲减退 appetite decreases

口渴 feel thirsty

多饮 drink water generously

体重增加 gain in weight

体重增加 8 千克 a 8 kilograms weight gain (gain 8 kilograms)

体重减轻 loss of weight (weight loss)

体重稳定不变 body weight is stable (unchanged, maintained)

睡眠障碍 somnipathy

睡眠不足 lack (want) of sleep

不易入睡 have trouble getting to sleep

睡眠过度 hypersomnia

嗜睡 somnolence (be fond of sleep)

失眠 have insomnia

睡眠差（好）sleep is poor (good)

消化不良 dyspepsia (have bad digestion)

大（小）便通畅 stool (urination) is easy and smooth (unobstructed, clear)

每日 2 次大便 have two stools daily

便秘（腹泻）constipation (diarrhea)

排尿困难 difficulty in micturition

尿频（急）frequency (urgency) of micturition

尿痛 micturition pain

少尿（无尿、多尿）oliguria (anuria, polyuria)

大便失禁 fecal incontinence

小便失禁 incontinence of urine

精神状态正常 orthophrenia (mental state is good)

精神不振 lassitude

精神紧张（抑郁）mental stress (depression)

168

（8）既往史、系统回顾和个人史 Past History, System Review and Personal History

　　1）既往史 Past History

- 无药物（食物）过敏史 no past history of allergy to drugs (food)
- 有……过敏史 have allergic history of
- 有肺结核接触史 there was contact history of lung tuberculosis
- 健康状况佳（差）health state was good (bad)
- 既往体健 be well (healthy) before
- 不详 not in detail (not quite clear)
- 否认既往心、肺疾病史 deny any history of prior heart and lung disease
- 10 年前曾患过…… suffered from...10 years ago
- 外伤史 trauma history
- 预防接种史 history of preventive inoculation

　　2）系统回顾 System Review

- 循环系统：气短、心悸、胸痛、咳嗽、咯血、水肿、晕厥

circulatory system: short of breath, palpitation, chest pain, cough、hemoptysis, edema, syncope.

- 呼吸系统：咳嗽、咳痰、呼吸困难、胸痛、盗汗、发热

respiratory system: cough, sputum, short of breath, chest pain, night sweating, fever.

- 消化系统：嗳气、反酸、腹胀、腹痛、腹泻、恶心和呕吐

alimentary system: belching, sour regurgitation, abdominal distension, abdominal pain, diarrhea, nausea and vomiting.

169

● 泌尿系统：排尿困难、尿频和尿急、尿痛、腹痛、水肿

urinary system: difficulty in micturition, frequency and urgency of micturition, painful micturition, abdominal pain, edema.

● 内分泌系统：心悸、怕热、多汗、烦渴、水肿、手抖、消瘦和肥胖

endocrine system: palpitation, heat intolerance, excessive sweating, polydipsia, edema, hand tremble, wasting and obesity.

● 造血系统：乏力、头晕、心悸、出血

hematopoietic system: fatigue, dizziness, palpitation, bleeding.

● 神经系统：头痛、晕厥、头晕和眩晕、失眠、偏瘫、失语

nervous system: headache, coma, dizziness and vertigo, insomnia, hemiplegia, aphasia.

● 运动系统：关节痛、麻木、跛行、瘫痪

motor system: joint pain, numbness, claudication, paralysis.

3）个人史 Personal History

● 出生于（出生地）was born in (birthplace)

● 出生后一直生活在……have lived in...since birth

● 曾（未曾）去过北方 have (deny having) been to the north

● 受教育程度（文盲、小学、中学、大学）educational level (illiterate, primary, middle, high grade)

● 从事……职业 be engaged in

● 卫生习惯和嗜好 health habit and special addiction

● 不洁性交（性行为）史 history of unsanitary intercourse

- 不吸烟 no smoking (not a smoker)
- 吸烟 10 年，每天 1 包 have smoked one packages of cigarette a day for 10 years
- 戒烟 give up (stop) smoking
- 不饮酒 no alcohol use
- 偶尔饮酒 drink little liquor occasionally
- 大量饮酒 drink heavily (too much)
- 偏食 food preference
- 无偏食 no likes or dislikes in food

（9）月经、婚姻、生育史和家族史 Menstrual, Marital and Childbearing History and Family History

1）月经史 Menstrual History

- 初潮年龄 age of menarche
- 月经周期 menstrual cycle
- 行经期 menstrual period
- 末次月经时间 last menstrual period (LMP)
- 月经正常 eumenorrhea (regular menses)
- 闭经年龄 age of menostasis
- 月经过多 menorrhagia (hypermenorrhea, menometrorrhagia)
- 月经过少 hypomenorrhea (scanty menstruation)
- 月经过频 polymenorrhea
- 痛经 dysmenorrhea (pain during the flow)
- 月经不调 menoxenia (irregular menses, menstrual disorder)
- 白带过多 profuse leukorrhea (whites)
- 经前水肿（疼痛）premenstrual edema (pain)
- 经量少（中、大）量 mild (moderate, heavy) menstrual blood

- 停经 pass the menopause at age...

  2）婚姻史 Marital History

- 未婚（已婚）single (married)
- 结婚年龄 age of wedding
- 配偶的健康状况 health status of partner (spouse)
- 近亲（非近亲）结婚 consanguineous (nonconsanguineous) marriage

  3）生育史 Childbearing History

- 妊娠（生育）次数和年龄 times and age of pregnancy (childbearing)
- 怀孕和生产次数 pregnancies and labors
- 人工（自然）流产次数 times of induced (spontaneous) abortion (miscarriage)
- 流产 miscarriage (abortion)
- 死胎 dead fetus
- 剖宫产 caesarean birth
- 子女数 number of children
- 早产 premature birth
- 足月产 term labor
- 自然分娩 be delivered normally and spontaneously (spontaneous labor)
- 产前（后）子痫 antepartum (postpartum) eclampsia
- 母乳喂养 breast feeding
- 人工喂养 artificial feeding
- 发育正常 normal development
- 发育异常（缺陷、畸形）developmental anomaly (defect, deformity)
- 发育迟缓 hypoevolutism

  4）家族史 Family History

- 遗传疾病 heredopathia (genetic disease)
- 遗传特征 hereditary feature

- 死因 cause of death
- 健康 be healthy (be in good healthy)
- 健在 be alive
- 无······家族史 no family history of...
- 死于······ die of...

3. 病 历 示 例

（1）内科病历 Medical Record Example of Internal Medicine

Acute myocardial infarction

Admission Notes

Name: ***	Birth place: ** Province
Gender: Male	Ethnic group: Chinese Han
Age: 60 years old	Date of Admission: Mar 21st 2019
Occupation: -	Date of Record: Mar 21st 2019
Marital status: Married	Source: Patient family member
Address: -	Reliability: Reliable

Chief Complaint: Sudden retrosternal pain for 2 hours

History of Present Illness:

2 hours before admission, with no inducing factors, the patient suffered from persistent crushing retrosternal chest pain suddenly, worst pain ever had, radiating to neck and left arm, accompanied with nausea, sweating and dizzy, without syncope. Glyceryl trinitrate（GTN）provided no relief. In emergency room of our hospital,

ECG: $V_1 \sim V_5$ ST segment elevation, T waves high. Echocardiography showed regional ventricular wall motion abnormality and the left ventricular ejection fraction (LVEF) was 52%. Troponin T was 2.79ng/ml. Then the patient was treated by aspirin 300mg and ticagrelor 180mg. Emergency coronary angiography outcome: LM (−), LAD 99% stenosis, LCX (−), RCA (−). The criminal vessel was revascularized by percutaneous transluminal coronary angioplasty (PTCA) and percutaneous coronary intervention (PCI). Then the patient was transferred into cardiovascular department. Since onset, his general state was good, foods could be taken as usual, defecation and urination are normal.

Past Medical History

Hypertension for 8 years, highest blood pressure 190/120mmHg, controlled to 140/90mmHg by Amlodipine 10mg q.d. p.o. Recently BP was not steady.

Diabetes mellitus for 8 years, controlled by Metformin 0.5g bid po and Acarbose 50mg t.i.d. p.o., controlling fasting blood glucose among $5 \sim 7$mmol/L and postprandial blood glucose among $9 \sim 11$mmol/L.

Dyslipidemia for 2 years, controlled by Atorvastatin.

2017-09-19 gastroscope: esophagitis, erosive gastritis, duodenal bulb inflammation.

He denied history of cerebrovascular disease, or exposure to viral hepatitis or TB. He denied history of operation, trauma or blood transfusion. No known drug or food allergies.

Systems review

Respiratory system: no cough, hemoptysis.

Circulatory system: no palpitation, edema.

Digestive system: no eructation, regurgitation, abdominal pain, diarrhea, jaundice, hematemesis, melena, or hematochezia.

Urinary and Genitourinary system: no waist pain and irritation syndrome of bladder.

Hematologic system: no paleness, bleeding, jaundice, hepatosplenomegaly or lymphadenopathy.

Endocrine system: no significant changes in character, no hyperpigmentation, hirsutism, or hyperhidrosis.

Musculoskeletal and neural system: no headache, vertigo, insomnia, convulsions, mental disorder, limb spasm or paralysis.

Social History

Born and living in ** Province. Denied tour to infected areas. Denied use of recreational medications. Cigarette use more than 30 years, 20~30 cigarettes every day. Denied exposure to toxins or radiation.

Marital history

He got married at the age of 27. His wife and a daughter were both in good state of health.

Family history

His parents have both dead, and his two brothers had been suffering from diabetes mellitus.

Physical Examination

T: 36.5℃　　P: 80 beats per minute　　R: 18 beats per minute　　BP: 110/70mmHg

Wt: 72kg　　Ht: 176cm　　BMI: 23.24 kg/m^2

General: Middle-aged man walking into the ward. Speaking complete sentences.

Skin: No jaundice, petechiae, skin lesions or fresh rash. No palmar erythema or spider angioma.

175

Lymph Nodes: No enlarged superficial lymph nodes.

HEENT:

Head: Hair of average texture. Scalp tender. Normocephalic/atraumatic (NC/AT).

Eyes: Conjunctiva pink; sclera anicteric.

Ears: Bilateral canal clear, TM with good cone of light.

Nose: Mucosa pink, septum midline. Bilateral frontal sinus tenderness.

Mouth: Oral mucosa pink and moist. Dentition good. Pharynx without exudates.

Neck: Neck supple. Trachea midline. Thyroid isthmus barely palpable, lobes not felt.

Breasts: Pendulous, symmetric. No masses. Nipples without discharge.

Thorax and Lungs:

Inspection: No use of accessory muscle.

Palpation: Tenderness over sternum and bilateral ribs. Thorax symmetric with good excursion. Lung resonant.

Percussion: No dullness to percussion.

Auscultation: Clear to auscultation bilaterally (CTAB). No rhonchi, wheezes, rales.

Cardiovascular:

Inspection: No jugular venous distension (JVD).

Palpation: Carotid upstrokes brisk, without bruits. Apical impulse palpable in the 5th left interspace, 8cm lateral to the midsternal line. No heaving apex impulse, thrill or pericardium friction rub could be palpated.

Percussion: Cardiac dullness shown below.

Right/cm	Intercostal Space(ICS)	Left/cm
2	II	2
3	III	4
4	IV	6
	V	7

Auscultation: Heart rate 72 beats per minite. Good S_1, S_2, no S_3 or S_4, with normal rhythm. No extra or abnormal heart sound, murmurs or pericardium friction sound. No gallops, or rubs.

Abdomen:

Inspection: flat.

Palpation & Percussion: No tenderness or distension (NT/ND). No rebound or guarding. No hepatosplenomegaly (HSM). Murphy sign (−). No costovertebral angle tenderness (CVAT). Shifting dullness sign (−).

Auscultation: Bowel sounds active.

Genitalia & Rectal: Normal distribution of pubic hair, without externalia malformation. No scar and ulcer.

Musculoskeletal: Spine with normal curve and no tenderness. No joint deformities. Good range of motion in hands, wrists, elbows, shoulders, spine, hips, knees, ankles. Warm and without edema or clubbing. Calves supple, nontender. Pulses brisk.

Neurology: Good muscle bulk and tone, pinprick, light touch, position sense, vibration and stereognosis intact. Right rapid alternating movements (RAMs), finger-to-nose test, heel-shin test slightly stupid. Romberg (−). Gait stable. Right biceps and triceps reflex active, bilateral patellar and achilles reflex active. Abdominal reflex (+), bilateral patellar clonus (−), bilateral ankle clonus (−), bilateral palmomental reflex (−), bilateral Hoffman sign (−), bilateral Babinski sign (−), bilateral Chaddock sign (−), bilateral Oppenheim sign (−), Gordon sign (−), neck supple, Kernig sign (−), Brudzinski sign (−), Lasegue sign (−).

Labs and Results

Echocardiography: LVEF 52%. Segmental wall motion abnormality. Secondary mitral regurgitation. Left atrial enlargement.

ECG: $V_1 \sim V_5$ ST segment elevation, T waves high.

Ultrasound: No obvious abnormality.

Myocardial injury markers: TNI 2.79ng/ml, MMB 1.5ng/ml, MYO 28.0ng/ml

BNP:403.0pg/ml

Initial Diagnosis: Acute extensive anterior myocardial infarction

Type 2 diabetes mellitus

Hypertension

Hyperlipemia

Assessment and Plan

Assessment: 60 years old male with acute extensive anterior myocardial infarction, type 2 diabetes mellitus, hypertension, hyperlipemia.

Problem/Plan-1

Problem: Acute extensive anterior myocardial infarction.

Plan: After surgery, monitoring vital signs, take antiplatelet drugs as aspirin 100mg q.d. and ticagrelor 90mg b.i.d..

Problem/Plan-2

Problem: Type 2 diabetes mellitus.

Plan: Take hypoglycemic drugs regularly, monitor blood sugar.

Problem/Plan-3

Problem: Hypertension.

Plan: Monitor blood pressure, take antihypertensive drugs(ACEI, β- blocker).

Problem/Plan-4

Problem: Hyperlipemia

Plan: Take Atorvastatin as usual.

Problem/Plan-5

Problem: Smoking.

Plan: Smoking cessation counseling, try to quit smoking.

（2）外科病历　Medical Record Example of Surgery

Thyroid Swelling (Goiter)

Admission Notes

Name: ***	Birth place: ** Province
Gender: Male	Ethnic group: Chinese Han
Age: 35 years old	Date of Admission: 11:00 a.m. 26th March 2019
Occupation: Music teacher	Date of Record: 11:00 a.m. 26th March 2019
Marital status: Married	Source: Self
Address: -	Reliability: Reliable

Chief Complaint: Noticed painless swelling in front of neck since 4 weeks

History of Present Illness:

The patient noticed a swelling in front of the neck while he was shaving about 4 weeks ago. He didn't sustain any trauma to the neck. Mr Zhang neither complained of difficulty in swallowing nor in breathing. He had a mild coryza one week prior to noticing the swelling, and it settled without any recourse to medication.

The swelling was painless and he didn't pay much attention to it but it gradually increased in size from the size of a pea to the size of an egg. Mr Zhang thus attended The First Affiliated Hospital of Sun Yat Sen University, where he was examined by Dr Wang, the famous endocrine surgeon and was diagnosed as having a thyroid swelling.

At the First Affiliated Hospital of Sun Yat Sen University, Mr Zhang undertook some basic blood test, had an ultrasound done and also had a thyroid scintigraphy scan. He was then referred to Dr Wang for further workup.

Past Medical History: Diagnosed with Diabetes Mellitus since 3 years. Currently, he is on Tab Metformin 500 mg bid po.

Past Surgical History: Operated for tonsillectomy at age 9 years and operated for appendectomy at age 13 years old. Uneventful post-surgical recovery.

Allergy History: No known history of allergy to any medication or food till date.

Personal History: Non-smoker. Occasional alcohol drinker. Drinks about 2~3 pegs of whiskey almost every alternate weekends. Non-vegetarian.

Family History: Father has diabetes mellitus

since 20 years and is on insulin injections. Mother is hypertensive but blood pressure is well controlled with medication and lifestyle changes. Has two elder brothers and one elder sister, all of whom in good health. No other specific disease in the family.

System Review:

Respiratory system: No cough, no fever, no haemoptysis, no dyspnoea.

Cardiopulmonary system: No chest pain, no palpitation, no diaphoresis, no orthopnoea, no paroxysmal nocturnal dyspnoea.

Gastrointestinal system: No abdominal pain, no vomiting, no bowel habit changes, no bleeding per rectum, no jaundice, no fever.

Urinary system: No urgency, no increased frequency of micturition, no dysuria, no low abdominal pain, no flank pain, no haematuria, no urinary retention, no dribbling of urine, no incontinence.

Endocrine system: Polyuria, polydipsia, no heat or cold intolerance, no striae, no diaphoresis, no change in weight.

Physical examination

Vital signs: T 37℃, HR 100/min, BP 140/87mmHg, RR 20/min.

Random blood sugar level 13 mmol/L, SpO_2 98% on air.

General: Normal development. Well nourished. No pallor. No icterus. No cyanosis. No pedal oedema.

Neck: Superficial lymph nodes not felt. Neck soft. No carotid bruit. Thyroid enlarged and not symmetrical. Non- tender swelling right side of thyroid, size 3cm×3cm. Thyroid swelling moves on deglutition. Trachea in midline. No engorgement of neck veins. Pharynx not congested. Absent tonsils.

Chest: Chest symmetrical. Bilateral chest equal air entry. Apex beat in 5th intercostal space at midclavicular line. Heart rate 100 beats per minite at rest. S_1 and S_2 heart sounds regular. No murmur heard.

Abdomen: Scaphoid appearance, soft, non-tender, non-distended, no guarding, no rigidity, no rebound tendernes. McBurney's incision scar for past appendectomy in right iliac fossa. Liver and spleen not appreciated on palpation. No obvious mass felt.

Laboratory Tests:

Thyroid function tests: Free T_3 90 ng/dl, TSH 1 mU/L.

ECG: Normal sinus rhythm, heart rate 100 beats per minites. No acute changes noted.

Chest X-Ray: Heart shadow looks normal. Bilateral lung fields appear clear.

X-Ray thoracic inlet: No obvious tracheal shift noted.

Ultrasound of the neck: Nodular swelling right thyroid lobe measuring 4.5cm×3.8cm in size. No increase in vascularity. No obvious enlarged lymph nodes noted.

Thyroid scintigraphy scan: Hypofunctioning nodule (cold nodule) right thyroid lobe.

Fine Needle Aspiration Cytology: Follicular adenoma. Excision biopsy is advised for confirmation.

Diagnosis:

Right Thyroid Lobe Cold Nodule

    (? Follicular adenoma)

    (Clinically euthyroid)

    Diabetes Mellitus

Signature: ****

（3）妇产科病历 Medical Record Example of Gynecology

Previa placenta

Admission Notes

Name: *** Birth place: Shanghai

Gender: Female Ethnic group: Chinese Han

Age: 38 years old Date of Admission: Nov 9th 2007

Occupation: Lawyer Date of Record: 09/11/2007

Marital status: Married Source: Patient herself

Address: No.20 Fenyang Road, Beijing Reliability: Reliable

Chief Complaint: 38-year-old gravidity 2 parity 10 01 female of 31^{+3} weeks gestation was admitted for vaginal bleeding.

History of Present Illness:

A 38-year-old gravidity 2 parity 10 01 female, whose LMP was April 2 and who has a pregnancy with an EGA of 31^{+3} weeks gestation, is brought to the emergency room by her husband. Complaining of vaginal spotting for the past two days. It has become heavier today, when she works up at 6:25 am to use the restroom she noted a sudden gush of bright red blood vaginally. She says that today's bleeding is more than a usual period and she became concerned when she passed a large clot. There is no mention of bleeding prior to any similar episode in the past with either pregnancy. She reports good fetal movement. She has had some contractions on and off, but nothing persistent. A review of her prenatal chart finds nothing remarkable other than a borderline high blood pressure from her first prenatal visit that has not required medication. She had an ultrasound to confirm pregnancy at 12 weeks. In addition, she has a positive h/o placenta previa at 20 weeks gestation with her current pregnancy determined by ultrasound. but none since.

When I enter the cubicle where she is resting, I notice an anxious, though pleasant, woman sitting upright on the gurney.

Prenatal Care: Peking University Third Hospital (PKU3), 1st visit Aug 6th 2007 with 10 total visits. Third trimester BPs were $100 \sim 104 / 68 \sim 84$ mmHg. Total weight gains 10 kg.

Pregnancy complicated by: Partial placenta previa

Prenatal Care Labs:

- Blood type: A+
- Rubella Ab titer: Immune
- VDRL test: Nonreactive (NR)
- Hemoglobin: 112 g/ L
- Hepatitis B: NR
- Cervical gonorrhea & Chlamydia culture: Negative
- Pap smear: Normal
- PPD skin test: Not done
- Sickle prep: Not done
- HIV test: NR
- RPR test: NR
- Quad screen: WNL(within normal limits)
- Group B strep: Not done
- Herpes: Denies
- Seizures: Denies
- Hepatitis C: NR
- OGTT: 90 / 170 / 150 /130mg/dl

- Non-invasive prenatal test: Low risk
- GBS: Not done
- Obstetrics ultrasound: Aug 23rd 2007, 20^{+3} weeks, ant. Placenta without previa, normal fetal survey

LMP: 02/04/2007

Expected date of confinement: Nov 2nd/2008

Past Medical History

Medication: Prenatal multivitamins daily. No regular medications, over-the-counter medications, or supplements. She has taken two days of the medications prescribed by the emergency room: Levaquin 500mg daily and Benzonatate 200mg t.i.d..

No history of hypertension or heart diseases. No history of diabetes or cerebrovascular disease. Patient denies history of hepatitis and tuberculosis. No history of allergies. No history of severe trauma and transfusion. Vaccinated regularly.

Allergies

No known drug allergies.

Systems review

Respiratory system: no cough, hemoptysis, chest pain or dyspnea.

Circulatory system: No palpitation, angina, or chest discomfort.

Digestive system: No nausea, vomiting, eructation, regurgitation, abdominal pain, diarrhea, jaundice, hematemesis, melena, or hematochezia.

Urinary and genitourinary system: No waist pain and irritation syndrome of bladder.

Hematologic system: No paleness, bleeding, jaundice, hepatosplenomegaly or lymphadenopathy.

Endocrine system: No polydipsia, polyuria and weight loss, no significant changes in character, no hyperpigmentation, hyper-trichiasis, or hyperhidrosis.

Musculoskeletal and neural system: no headache, dizziness, vertigo, insomnia, convulsions, mental disorder, limb spasm and paralysis.

Social History

Born and grown up in Shanghai. Patient lives in **Rd with her husband and her child. She denies having a job and states that her husband helps her with finances. No use of recreational medications. The patient denies tobacco or I.V. drug use, but reports occasional EtOH use with last time in April. No recent travel or sick contacts.

Menstrual, Marital and Childbearing history

The menarche: At 13 years old.

Menses: Regular 28 days cycles with 4 days duration menses, heavy flow first two days and becomes gradually lighter toward end of menses.

Contraception hx: Denies use of barrier or hormonal methods.

LMP: 02/04/2007

Married at the age of 28. G_1P_1. 2002: Caesarean-section 2ary to non-reassuring fetal heart tracings. Boy, weight 3 500g. Her husband and her son are both in good state of health.

Family history

No family history of lung disease, hypertension or clotting disorders. No family history of DM or stroke. No family history of nervous or mental diseases. Mother died at 92 of "old age." Father died in a traffic accident, no chronic health problems. The patient has two healthy siblings.

Physical Examination

T: 36.5℃   P: 76 beats per minute   R: 18 beats per minute   BP: 180/120mmHg

Wt: 64kg   Archive weight: 51kg   Ht: 166cm   BMI: 23.23kg/m^2

General: Middle-aged woman is lying in the gurney; speaking complete sentences, anxious, though pleasant.

Skin: Pink, cool and dry. No jaundice, petechiae, skin lesions or fresh rash. No palmar erythema or spider angioma. Conceivable edema across the whole body.

Lymph Nodes: Small (<1cm), soft, nontender, and mobile tonsillar and posterior cervical nodes bilaterally. No axillary or epitrochlear nodes. Several small inguinal nodes bilaterally, soft and nontender.

HEENT:

Head: Hair of average texture. Scalp tender. Normocephalic/ atraumatic (NC/AT).

Eyes: Conjunctiva pink, sclera anicteric.

Ears: Bilateral canal clear, TM with good cone of light.

Nose: Mucosa pink, septum midline. Bilateral frontal sinus tenderness.

Mouth: Oral mucosa pink and moist. Dentition good. Pharynx without exudates.

Neck: Neck supple. Trachea midline. Thyroid isthmus barely palpable, lobes not felt.

Breasts: Pendulous, symmetric. No masses, nipples without discharge.

Thorax and Lungs:

Inspection: No use of accessory muscle.

Palpation: Tenderness over sternum and bilateral ribs. Thorax symmetric with good excursion. Lung resonant.

Percussion: No dullness to percussion.

Auscultation: Clear to auscultation bilaterally (CTAB). No rhonchi, wheezes, rales.

Cardiovascular

Inspection: No jugular venous distension (JVD).

Palpation: Carotid upstrokes brisk, without bruits. Apical impulse palpable in the 5th left interspace, 8cm lateral to the midsternal line. No heaving apex impulse, thrill or pericardium friction rub could be palpated.

Percussion: The border of cardiac is not enlarged. Cardiac dullness shown below.

Right /cm	Intercostal Space(ICS)	Left /cm
2.5	II	2
2.5	III	4
3	IV	6
	V	8

The centerline of the left clavicle is located 8cm left of the front midline.

Auscultation: Heart rate 90 beats per minite. Good S_1, S_2, no S_3 or S_4, with normal rhythm. No extra or abnormal heart sound, murmurs or pericardium friction sound. No gallops, or rubs.

Abdomen:

Inspection: Universal abdominal bulge. No ventral

stripe, chromatists, spider angioma and hernia observed. Cesarean section scar is at the lower abdomen.

Palpation & Percussion: No tenderness or distension (NT/ND). No rebound or guarding. Murphy sign (−). No costovertebral angle tenderness (CVAT).

Auscultation: Bowel sounds heard in all 4 quadrants.

Genitalia & Rectal: Normal distribution of pubic hair, without external malformation. No scar and ulcer.

Musculoskeletal: Spine with normal curve and no tenderness. No joint deformities. Good range of motion in hands, wrists, elbows, shoulders, spine, hips, knees, ankles. Warm and without edema or clubbing. Calves supple, nontender. Pulses brisk.

Neurology: Good muscle bulk and tone. pinprick, light touch, position sense, vibration and stereognosis intact. Right rapid alternating movements (RAMs), finger-to-nose test, heel-shin test slightly stupid. Romberg (−). Gait stable. Right biceps and triceps reflex active, bilateral patellar and Achilles reflex active. Abdominal reflex (+), bilateral patellar clonus (−), bilateral ankle clonus (−). Bilateral palm-omental reflex (−), bilateral Hoffman sign (−), bilateral Babinski sign (−), bilateral Chadlock sign (−), bilateral Oppenheim sign (−), Gordon sign (−). Neck supple. Kernig sign (−), Brudzinski sign (−), LA segue sign (−).

Obstetric examination

Abdominal girth: 93cm.

Height of fundus: 29cm, slightly irregular in contour but nontender.

Fetal present: head present.

Fetal position: LOA.

Fetal heart rate(FHR): 137 beats per minute

Pelvis: 23-27-19-9cm

Vaginal exam: Speculum exam reveals no active bleeding from the cervix, although there is evidence of old blood in the vaginal vault. The cervical os is closed. No lesions are present in the vagina or on the vulva.

The external monitor reveals uterine irritability, but no discrete contractions are seen.

- Non-stress test (NST): baseline FHR of 137 beats per minute, reactive with accelerations and frequent variability.

Labs and Results

Date of exam	Tests	Results	Institution
2007.11.09	Blood RT	Hb 100g/L; PLT 136× 10^9/L	PKU3.
2007.11.09	Urine RT	uric protein (−); occlude blood: (−)	PKU3.
2007.11.09	Obstetrics Ultrasound	BPD 78mm; HC 259mm; AC 238mm; FL 51mm; Degree of placental maturity: Ⅱ; placenta with partial coverage of cervical internal os. fetal heartbeat and fetal movement seen. amniotic fluid depth: 64mm. Umbilical A : PI : 0.87; R_2 0.59; S/D 2.46; FHR 137beats per minute	PKU3.

continue

Date of exam	Tests	Results	Institution
2007.11.09	Serum potassium	3.9mmol/L	PKU3.
2007.11.09	Scr	86μmol/L	PKU3.
2007.11.09	Liver function	ALT 25U/L ; AST 30U/L	PKU3.

Initial Diagnosis: G_2P_1, pregnancy 31^{+3}weeks, LOA

Placenta previa.

Scarred uterus

Anemia

Assessment and Plan

Assessment: A 38-year-old woman who has presented to the emergency room with vaginal bleeding. Patient is 38-year-old gravidity 2 parity 10 01 female of 31^{+3} weeks gestation. The external monitor reveals uterine irritability, but no discrete contractions are seen. NST: Baseline FHR of 137 beats per minute, reactive with accelerations and frequent variability. The patient's vital sign is stable. Sonographic evaluation of placental location is partial coverage of cervical internal os. with rolling out placenta previa.

There are multiple causes of vaginal bleeding on the third trimester of pregnancy. Thoughtful, prompt evaluation and management are necessary to reduce the threat to the lives of the mother and fetus. The differential diagnosis should include:

1) Obstetric causes. a. Placental: Placental previa, placental abruption, circumvallate placenta, placenta accrete, placenta increta, placenta percreta. b. Maternal: Uterine rupture, clotting disorders. c. Fetal: Fetal vessel rupture.

2) Non-obstetric causes. a. Cervical: Severe cervicitis, polyps, benign/malignant neoplasms. b. Vaginal: Lacerations, varices, benign/malignant neoplasms. c. Other: Hemorrhoids, bleeding disorder, abdominal/pelvic trauma. The average gestational age at the time of first bleeding episode is $29\sim30$ weeks. Although bleeding may be substantial, it is usually spontaneous.

Based on the patient's negative history for 2nd trimester vaginal bleeding, premature labor, premature rupture of membrane, closed cervix and lack of labor contractions, it is likely that her vaginal bleeding is a sign of premature labor. The patient has a positive history of placenta previa with this pregnancy in addition to a previous Caesarean-section which leads to suspect vaginal bleeding caused by partial placenta previa. U/S/ revealed no signs of placenta accrete, increta, or percreta. The best medical approach for her pregnancy's gestational age is expectant management in the hospital with bed rest, with details discussed below.

Problem/Plan-1

Problem: Vaginal bleeding in placenta previa is not painless and may also stop as abruptly as it had begun. When the placenta is unable to stretch to accommodate the shape of the cervix, bleeding will occur suddenly that could frighten the woman.

Plan:

1) Hospitalize patient and initiate bed rest for at least 5 days for evaluation.

2) Assess maternal and fetal status by monitoring maternal vital signs and NST for fetal heart function daily for hospital stay duration.

3) Ultrasound uterus and evaluate fetal growth, movement, and heart functioning, as well as placental location and implantation status.

Problem/Plan-2

Problem:

Risk of preterm labor: In placenta previa, vaginal bleeding appears to arise from disruption of the placental implantation site as the lower uterine segment develops. It is unclear whether uterine contractions play a role, as only 20% of women with placenta previa have uterine activity at the time of vaginal bleeding. It is difficult to determine whether these women have true preterm labor, because digital examination of the cervix to document cervical dilatation is impossible.

Plan:

1) Discuss with patient the advantages and disadvantages of tocolytic therapy. Magnesium sulfate administration with close observation of flexion of knee, respiratory rate and urine. Control hypertension with Labetalol or Nitroglycerin.

2) Cautious evaluation of the maternal and fetal complications and take action correspondingly.

3) Use corticosteroids to accelerate fetal lung maturity. Delivery at an appropriate time.

4) Arrange pediatric consultation if preterm birth is anticipated.

Problem/Plan-3

Problem:

Anemia: Admission labs show hemoglobin at 100g/L, with MCV of 89.5, so this anemia is normocytic. The patient denies any history of anemia when questioned, and was not dizzy, pale, or fatigued despite of repeated vaginal bleeding.

Plan:

Check Fe panel, hemoccult stools, monitor Hb, iron supplement to correct anemia.

Problem/Plan-4

Problem:

High risk of thromboembolic: The patient is admitted to hospital and has a period of bed rest. She is at third trimester of pregnancy.

Plan:

Initiate measures to prevent thrombosis e.g. wearing knee high compression stockings continuously until fully mobile. Promote frequent leg exercises until fully mobile.

Problem/Plan-5

Problem:

Anxious: The patient appears very anxious about her pregnancy and that she has a lot of questions about why she had a placenta previa.

Plan:

Arrange for 'Parent Education' staff to provide antenatal education for her. Advise the patient with placenta previa to avoid penetrative sexual intercourse. Vaginal and rectal examinations should be avoided.

Signature: ****

4. 其他医疗文书 Other Medical Documents

（1）病程记录 Progress Notes

Progress notes are official documents to record

a patient's details throughout the whole process of treatment during hospitalization. They are included in the patient's medical record for the purpose of recording as proof that the patient has been regularly contacted, assessed and treated, providing the clinical reasoning behind and guiding the other health care providers involved on understanding the patient's condition so as to provide the most accurate treatment. Therefore, progress notes should be organized in a concise and clear manner and should be documented timely. The well-accepted structured format of progress note is SOAP (A-Subjective, O-Objective, A-Assessment, P-Plans).

Progressive Note

8:00 am, Feb. 27th, 2019, POD#1 (Post Operative Day 1) after right up lobectomy

Subjective:

The patient complains of mild chest pain, nausea and coughing up blood, no shortness of breath, no vomiting during the night, "feeling better this morning".

Objective:

Vitals Signs: T 36.9℃, BP 120/80mmHg, HR 90 beats per minute, RR 18, SpO_2 100% on 2L/m NC (Nasal Cannula).

Chest tube drainage: Unobstructed chest drainage tube leads to pale bloody fluid 120 ml, no blood clot, no air leakage.

Urine volume: 1 500ml.

Wound: well-approximated, no erythema, C/D(Clean and Dry).

Lungs: Breath sounds clear, slightly decreased on the right side.

CV (Cardiovascular): Clear to auscultation and percussion.

Abdomen: oft, ND/NT (no distended/no tenderness), normal active BS (bowel sound).

EXT (extremities): Warm, no edema.

Labs:

CBC (complete blood count): WBC 9.4×10^9/L, Hb 10.8g/L, Hct 31.4%, PLT 319×10^9/L.

CHEM (chemistry): Na^+ 138mmol/L, K^+ 4.9mmol/L, Cl^- 106mmol/L, HCO_3^- 27mmol/L, BUN 26mmol/L, Cr 8μmol.

Bedside CR (chest radiograph): Chest tube well positioned, no collapsing of lung, no pleural effusion, no pneumothorax.

Assessment:

Post-operative day 1 for VATS lobectomy, recovering well.

Pain control adequate.

Transient nausea appears secondary to anesthetics administration, clinically at this time he voices feeling well.

Plan:

Remove chest tube.

OOB (get out of bed) and ambulate, increase activity level in the afternoon.

Advance diet.

Stop of antibiotics.

（2）会诊申请 Consultation Request Note

It's not uncommon that the diagnosis or treatment of doubtful cases requires the joint effort of multiple physicians or disciplines. Accurate communication between the referral physician and the consultation physician paves the way for effective communication and produces favorable outcomes for timely access to patient care. A consultation request note should contain the patient's information, clinical condition. The existing problem and pertaining investigation results should be addressed, and the reason and purpose of consultation be clarified.

Consultation Request Note

Patient data:

Name: Li Ming　Case Number:　259622　Bed Number: 10F-1

From:　Dr. Ye, Dept. of General Thoracic Surgery

To: Dr. Du, Dept. of Cardiology

Reason for request: Preoperative assessment

Provisional diagnosis: Right upper lobe lung cancer, cT1N0M0 - stage Ia1

Operation planned: VATS right upper lobectomy and systemic lymphadenectomy

Clinical information:

Briefly, the patient is a 65-year-old gentleman with history of smoking >30 pack- year, 1cm solid nodule found on CT screening. He denied coughing up blood. He was admitted to the hospital and diagnosed with lung cancer, planned for operation.

The patient had a history of hypertension for 10 years. He denied other systemic diseases, denied chest pain on exertion. The patient had no shortness of breath or weakness. He is able to climb 5 flights of stairs without stopping.

Recent medication: None

His ECG revealed sinus rhythm, and he did rule out for myocardial infarction with serial cardiac enzymes. BNP normal.

Echocardiography demonstrated enlarged left ventricle diameter: end-diastolic 70mm and end-systolic 63 mm, moderate mitral regurgitation, severely depressed global function with EF 27%.

Pulmonary function tests: FEV_1 1.86 (82% of predicted) and DLCO 9.6 (72%).

Given the patient's clinical stability on one hand and measured poor EF on the other hand, I am requesting cardiology evaluation of the suitability of general anesthesia and right upper lobe lobectomy for this patient.

Thank you for the assistance.

Signature of referring physician

Date

（3）出院小结 Discharge Summary

Discharge summary is a general report of a patient's details of examinations, diagnoses and the whole progress of treatment during hospitalization. It also provides professional instructions to a patient and his (or her) family, and also severs as written communicating to the post-discharge medical care. Precise discharge summaries are essential for patient care continuity and safety. The document would ideally be ready to go with the discharged patient.

The documented information should be concise, but the following items are the most important components which should be contained in a high-quality discharge summary: patient information, diagnosis (both admission and discharge), reasons for hospitalization, significant findings, treatment provided, discharge condition, post-discharge instructions.

Discharge Summary

Patient data:

Name: Li Ming   Case Number: 259276

Bed Number: 10F-2

Sex: Male   Age: 68

Discharge department: Department of General Thoracic Surgery.

Date of admission: Feb 22th, 2019.

Date of discharge: Feb 30th, 2019.

Admission diagnosis:

1. Right upper lobe nodule.

2. Hypertension.

Discharge diagnosis:

1. Right lung upper lobe adenocarcinoma, pT1N0M0, Stage Ia.

2. Hypertension.

3. HFrEF (Heart Failure with Reduced Ejection Fraction), Stage B, NYHA Class 1.

Reasons for hospitalization, and hospital course:

The patient is a 68-year-old male with a past medical history of hypertension was found to have a nodule in his upper lobe of lung when receiving screening chest CT scan. He denied coughing or coughing up blood. He had a smoking history >20 pack- year, The patient had no shortness of breath on exertion, no headaches, no bone or joint pain, no weight loss.

Well developed, well nourished. Afebrile, no

palpable neck or supraclavicular lymphadenopathy. Breathing movement fair and symmetrical. Lungs clear to auscultation and percussion. Regular heart rhythm, no murmur or gallop. Extremities without cyanosis or clubbing.

Laboratory data:

Labs: CBC, serum chemistries were normal, blood type: Type O, RH(+).

Chest CT with contrast: solid nodule (1cm in diameter) confined to the apex segment of right lung, the boundary is irregular and spiculate, partial pleural pulled, without hilar or mediastinal lymphadenopathy. Remarkably enlarged cardiac contour with coronary artery calcifications.

MRI Head: No cerebral metastasis was detected.

PET-CT: Hypermetabolic activity in the known right upper lobe nodule, no hypermetabolic mediastinal or hilar lymph nodes are noted. No worrisome hypermetabolic actviey is seen within the neck, abdomen, pelvis, or bone.

ECG revealed sinus rhythm.

Cardiac Echo: Echocardiography demonstrated enlarged left ventricle with end-diastolic 70mm and end-systolic 63 mm, depressed left ventricle function with EF of 27%, moderate mitral regurgitation.

Pulmonary function tests: FEV_1 1.72 (80% of predicted) and DLCO 9.8 (73%).

Important consultation:

A severely depressed left ventricle function and low EF (27%) was measured with cardiac echo, he was referred to department of cardiology for pre-operation assessment. Given the well preserved physical activity and compensated heart function, albeit depressed left ventricle function, the patient was recommended to receive operation with no further testing/intervention.

Pathological findings:

Right upper lobe adenocarcinoma, grade 2, metastasis negative for stations 2R, 4R, 7, 8, 9, 10, 11, 12 lymph nodes.

Immunohistochemical stains: TTF-1(+), CK7(−), ki67 positive rate 37%, napsin A(+), p63(+), CK5/6(+).

Treatment provided:

The patient received VATS right upper lobe lobectomy and systemic lymphadenectomy under general anesthesia on Feb. 24th, 2019. The procedure was completed without complications and the patient experienced an uneventful recovery.

Complications: None

Discharge condition:

T 36.9℃, RR 17, BP 130/70mmHg, HR 80 beats per minute.

Good general status, able to ambulate without difficulty. No shortness of breath. Surgical wounds heal clean and dry.

Discharge medication: Amlodipine Besylate 5mg orally once daily.

Discharge instructions:

Return to the emergency room if: You cannot think clearly, your lips or nails look blue or pale, you have a headache or dizziness, you have more swelling in your face, arms, neck, or chest.

Early postoperative check-up in two weeks (obtain final pathological report and check surgical wound healing)

Cardiology out-patient follow-up for HFrEF.

Long-term follow up advised (every 4 months for the first two years followed by annual check)

Adopt a physically active lifestyle

Do not smoke.

Signature of physician

（4）病例讨论 Case Discussion

Case discussion is one of the important teaching activities to train students in clinical diagnosis, treatment and prognosis decision-making during graduation internship. The purpose is to train interns to learn the knowledge and experience of medical seniors, outstanding physicians and students, to learn the ability to analyze and solve clinical problems, and to exercise self-study and oral expression skills. The implementation of the clinical medical record discussion is based on a heuristic discussion teaching approach that embodies the interaction between teachers and students. It is a new teaching mode with students as the main body, teachers as the medium and knowledge as the object. Discussions on clinical cases include: typical cases, difficult cases, deaths, etc. Clinical teaching case discussions (teaching rounds) in each ward are usually scheduled 1~2 times a month.

Preparation for the Teaching Ward：

1) Host of the teaching round: An attending physician or above.

2) Case preparation: The teacher selects representative typical cases with teaching significance (the disease is relatively stable, the medical history is typical,

the symptoms and signs are obvious, and the diagnosis is basically clear). The case should be a common disease, frequently-occurring disease, and patients with significant curative effect after treatment.

3) Medical data preparation: Preparation of cases and other related auxiliary examinations, such as electrocardiogram, X-ray, CT, etc., the content is informative and complete.

4) Patient preparation: Get the patient's consent in advance, and get their cooperation.

5) Teaching preparation: The attending doctor should inform the intern case and bed number in advance. Before the teaching ward, the attending physician should fully understand the patient's recent situation and have a thorough understanding of the patient's medical history, physical signs, auxiliary examination, diagnosis, treatment and prognosis. Familiar with basic theory, basic knowledge and basic skills.

6) Student preparation: Familiarize with the patient's condition in advance, review the medical record and view the theoretical knowledge related to the case. The intern who is responsible for the bed uses the necessary instruments (check trolleys or trays) for teaching, including sphygmomanometers, thermometers, stethoscopes, hammers, flashlights, scales, tongue depressors, cotton swabs, pens, hand sanitizers, etc.

Sample of Teaching Ward:

Director: Dr. Zhang	**Resident:** Dr. Lee
Attending physician: Dr. Yang	**Interns:** Dr. Zhao
Chief resident: Dr. Liu	**medical student:** Dr. Wang

Dr. Liu: Good morning everyone, case discussion begins. Today we focus the ectopic pregnancy. Where the embryo is implemented outside the uterus, collectively referred to as ectopic pregnancy. It is one of the common acute abdomens in obstetrics and gynecology. When the tubal pregnancy is aborted or ruptured, it can cause severe bleeding and shock. If it is not diagnosed or actively rescued, it can be life-threatening. First of all, I would like to invite Dr. Lee present the case.

Dr. Lee: 25-year-old woman who has presented to the emergency room complaining of vaginal spotting for the past two days, and which has become heavier today. She says that today bleeding is more than a usual period and she became concerned when she passed a large clot. When I enter the cubicle where she is resting, I notice an anxious, though pleasant, woman sitting upright on the gurney. She denies fever, chills, abdominal pain or cramping. She says that she has been urinating more frequently than usual, without pain, and notes fatigue that she attributes to stress at her work as a pastry chef. She is unable to tell me when her last menstrual period was since she has had irregular menses since puberty, often with two to three-month gaps between periods. She has never been pregnant. She tells me that she and her boyfriend, who plan to marry in the next year, use condoms for contraception. She has never been diagnosed with a sexually transmitted infection. She gave no history suggestive of intake of ovulation induction drugs. Her general appearance is that of a well-developed female with 69kg and 160cm tall. On physical exams, her vital signs are stable and she is not orthostatic. Arterial blood pressure (BP) was 100/60mmHg, pulse was 88 beats per minite and body temperature was measured as 36.5℃. An examination of her abdomen reveals normal bowel sounds, Lower abdomen tenderness, rigidity and guarding were present. Speculum exam reveals no active bleeding from the cervix, although there is evidence of old blood in the vaginal vault. The cervical os is closed. No lesions are present in the vagina or on the vulva. Bimanual exam reveals a slightly enlarged and globular uterus in mid-position; the left adnexa revealed tenderness with a palpable masses. The next steps I should to assess this patient in below: Evaluate for pregnancy, determine whether pregnancy is intrauterine and determine whether pregnancy is viable.

Dr. Yang: In a woman of childbearing age who presents with an unknown last menstrual period, it is important to determine her pregnancy status. A history of irregular menses is not uncommon, especially in teenagers or in overweight women and, in this setting, a qualitative urine pregnancy test is crucial. The diagnosis of pregnancy should not be made on nonspecific signs and symptoms. Dr. Zhao, would you tell us about the sign and symptom of pregnancy?

Dr. Zhao: Signs and symptoms of pregnancy include the flowing: At first the history such as: missed periods, fatigue, nausea and vomiting, breast tenderness, urinary frequency, the second is physical exam: Softening and enlargement of the uterus, congestion and bluish discoloration of the vagina, softening of the cervix。

Dr. Yang: What is the differential diagnosis for this patient? Which specific symptoms and signs does this patient have that are suspicious for an ectopic pregnancy?

Dr. Wang: Differential diagnoses for vaginal bleeding in a young lady includes ectopic pregnancy, incomplete, completed, or missed abortion, threatened abortion, ovarian cyst, adnexal torsion, pelvic inflammatory disease, endometriosis, appendicitis and gastrointestinal etiologies, urinary tract infections or stones. The physical examination is important in ruling out adnexal masses or pain that indicate a possible ectopic pregnancy. Uterine size is a clue to the presence of an intrauterine pregnancy, though fibroids (leiomyomata) or adenomyosis can also cause uterine enlargement. Typically, pregnancy size is given in terms of the estimated gestational age or the size of fruit, with a six to eight-week size uterus the size of a large orange, 12~14 weeks that of a grapefruit, and 14~16 weeks the size of a cantaloupe. A 12-week size uterus can be felt at the symphysis pubis and a 20-week size pregnancy reaches the level of the umbilicus. The accepted norm for pregnancy dating in the absence of a firm last menstrual period date is the ultrasound.

Signs and physical positive findings include in this patient: abdominal tenderness, adnexal tenderness, normal uterine size and adnexal mass(Figure 3-1).

Dr. Yang: Very good, what risk factors predispose patients to ectopic pregnancy and which of these risk factors does this patient have (indicated with an *)?

Dr. Liu: ①Previous ectopic pregnancy (approx 10 times increase). ②History of pelvic inflammatory disease, gonorrhea, or chlamydia infections. ③History of previous gyn or abdominal surgery. ④Sterilization

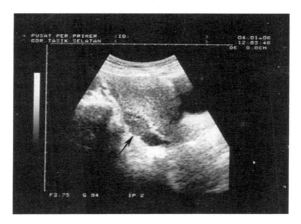

Figure 3-1　transvaginal sonographic images:
Normal uterine size and adnexal mass

failure. ⑤Endometriosis. ⑥Congenital uterine malformation. ⑦Older age (35～44 years old are 3 times higher risk than younger women). Often, diagnosing and managing a patient with an ectopic pregnancy can be difficult. Knowledge of the risk factors can heighten the clinician's suspicion and may determine the direction of the investigation. Now, another question is which the most important test to do next in order to narrow down our diagnosis?

Dr. Lee: Human chorionic gonadotropin (hCG) is the most important test. Sometimes skipped which can lead to mortality or morbidity. A blood sample (for CBC to determine whether anemia is present in the setting of vaginal bleeding) and a urine specimen (for urinalysis and urine pregnancy test) should be obtained. Urine pregnancy tests measure hCG and standard tests become positive approximately 4 weeks following the first day of the last menstrual period.

Many emergency rooms have access to laboratory facilities that can give rapid serum quantitative hCG (qhCG) results and this can be important in the setting of a threatened miscarriage or possible ectopic pregnancy where the measurement of qhCG levels over time can assist in making the diagnosis.

The patient's CBC and UA are normal with a hemoglobin concentration of 10.0 g/dl and hematocrit of 29.1%. The urine pregnancy test is positive. This patient's hCG level was 1 450U/L. What next tests could be helpful in making a more definitive diagnosis?

Dr. Wang: The ultrasound will help determine whether the pregnancy is viable and whether it is intrauterine or not. A rule of thumb is the earlier the ultrasound, the more reliable as far as dating. In practice, many ultrasounds are performed at about 16~20 weeks gestation, which ensures both accurate dating and the opportunity of evaluating the fetal for developmental abnormalities. The later in pregnancy an ultrasound is performed, the less reliable is its dating ability, due to the variance is fetal size with advancing gestation. In very early pregnancy and particularly in obese women, a transvaginal ultrasound may be necessary to identify the pregnancy and fetal cardiac activity. Otherwise, trans-abdominal ultrasonography may be performed. Fetal cardiac activity visualized on ultrasound confirms viability and should be present when the embryo is 5mm in length or more (by TV U/S, corresponds to approximately 5 weeks GA). A ultrasonographic scanning by the emergency physician during the pelvic exam revealed an empty uterus with an endometrium 15mm thick and a left adnexal mass of 3cm×4cm×4cm. Ectopic pregnancy was identified.

Dr. Yang: Initial to see if level is >1 500U/L so that lack of intrauterine pregnancy on transvaginal ultrasound can lead to a high suspicion of extra-uterine pregnancy. This patient's hCG level was 1 450U/L, absence of a period of amenorrhoea. A detailed menstrual history is important and any sudden change of menstrual pattern should alert us to think of the possibility of tubal ectopic pregnancy even in the absence of a clear period of amenorrhoea in women in the reproductive age group. In some case, there are no clinical symptoms. Up to 30% of women with ectopic pregnancy will have symptoms similar to gastrointestinal and genitourinary disorder, such as anal flatulence, nausea, metastatic lower abdominal pain. So different diagnosis is very important. I would like to invite Director Zhang comment on pitfalls in diagnosis of EP and ruptured ectopic.

Dr. Zhang: EP is one of the most common Gynecological emergencies. EP occurs in 2% of all pregnancies, the myriad of locations have a hierarchy of prevalence as well as associated mortality and morbidity. The most common location of the ectopic pregnancy continues to be fallopian tubes (accounting for roughly 95% of all ectopic pregnancies). It turns out that we're missing the diagnosis more than we'd like to admit. I would like this teaching around ectopic pregnancy so that we can improve our diagnostic skills for this potentially life threatening diagnosis. When you suspect EP, you should do the follow: ①Ruling out ectopic pregnancy based on β-hCG level. There is no β-hCG level or series of β-hCG levels at which ectopic can be ruled out. The traditional teaching of a β-hCG level <1 000 ruling out ectopic can distract from making the diagnosis of ruptured ectopic in a timely manner. Ectopic pregnancy may present with rising, falling or plateau, or even zero β-hCG levels. ②Relying on a urine ß-hCG in early pregnancy. Urine β-hCG is unreliable (false negatives early in pregnancy). Always obtain serum β-hCG. ③Assuming low risk of ectopic pregnancy in a patient with no identifiable risk factors. The majority of patients with ectopic pregnancy have no identifiable risk factors (tubal surgery or known abnormality, previous ectopic, PID/STI, current IUD, history of infertility, IVF). ④Assuming low risk of ruptured ectopic pregnancy based on normal vital signs. Patient with ruptured ectopic may present with normal vitals or even with bradycardia despite a litre or 2 of blood in their bellies. Normal vitals do not rule out ruptured ectopic pregnancy. ⑤Assuming that a patient taking methotrexate for known ectopic pregnancy presenting with abdominal pain has a low risk for rupture. The risk of rupture when patients are being treated with methotrexate for ectopic esp if relative contraindications to methotrexate (6% failure rate: level of ß-hCG correlates with failure rate. guidelines suggest only trying methotrexate with ß-hCG <5 000). ⑥Forgoing or delaying a transvaginal ultrasound to rule out ectopic based on history physical and ß-hCG in first trimester bleed or first trimester abdominal pain. T1 bleed or pain should get a TV ultrasound in ED as no combination of history, physical, beta or progesterone that can rule out ectopic or ruptured ectopic.

Dr. Yang: What would our next step in management be? What other counseling or advice you need to discuss with this patient?

Dr. Liu: Once the diagnosis is entertained, the first step is to determine whether the patient is hemodynamically stable. The possibility of ectopic pregnancy was explained to her and she was admitted immediately to our hospital as she could collapse as a result of haemoperitoneum. I will be able to discuss various treatment options with the patient. General ectopic pregnancy management options are: surgical (salpingectomy or salpingotomy), medical(methotrexate injection) and expectant (wait and see). Several weeks of follow-up are required with each treatment. In this case, the patient is stable, with pulse and blood pressure within normal limits, and there is no heavy bleeding or severe pain, and there are no signs of dizziness or fainting, and the ectopic is early (ß-hCG levels < 3 000 U/L), so she should take methrotrexate.

This drug stops cells from growing, which ends the pregnancy. The pregnancy then is absorbed by the body over 4~6 weeks. This does not require the removal of the fallopian tube. Methrotrexate medical treatment requirements: ①Hemodynamically stable. ②No fetal heart beat seen outside of the uterus. ③Ectopic gestation that is not too big (usually <3.5cm). Cooperative patient who will be sure to return for follow-up and serial hCGs and will report increased pain.

If the patient is unstable, bleeding heavily, in severe pain or have signs of dizziness or fainting, I will probably

211

suggest an exploratory emergency surgical operation. the patient requires esuscitation, two large-bore I.V.'s were started, the patient was cross-matched for blood. The most common is laparoscopy or laparotomy. If her fallopian tube is damaged, she may have to remove it as well.

Dr. Zhang: Ectopic pregnancy is a condition of immense gynecological importance. Ectopic pregnancies could be asymptomatic, especially before rupture. When ruptured, symptoms could be acute or subacute, and as such is a true medical emergency. Early diagnosis and appropriate management may prevent serious adverse outcomes and potentially improve subsequent fertility.

Patients with ruptured ectopic pregnancy could present with signs of shock, including hypotension, tachycardia, and rebound tenderness. When a pregnant patient presents with first-trimester bleeding or abdominal pain, you should consider ectopic pregnancy as a possible cause. The patient history, physical examination, and imaging with transvaginal ultrasonography can usually confirm the diagnosis. Pregnancy tests were used as supportive diagnostic investigations, with diagnosis confirmed by trans-abdominal ultrasound scan.

When ultrasonography does not clearly identify the pregnancy location, the physician must determine whether the pregnancy is intrauterine (either viable or failing) or ectopic. Failure to visualize an intrauterine pregnancy when β-hCG is above the discriminatory level suggests ectopic pregnancy. In addition to single measurements of β-hCG levels, serial levels can be monitored to detect changes. β-hCG values in approximately 99% of viable intrauterine pregnancies increase by about 50% in 48 hours. After an ectopic pregnancy has been confirmed, treatment options include medical, surgical, or expectant management. For patients who are medically unstable or experiencing life-threatening hemorrhage, a surgical approach is indicated, the same times, supportive treatment including I.V. fluids, MAST suits, oxygen, bed rest and transfusion as need can often be effective management of these patients. For others, management should be based on patient preference after discussion of the risks, benefits, and monitoring requirements of all approaches.

That is all for today, thanks everybody.

（5）常用医嘱和缩写 Commonly Used Medical Orders and Abbreviations

Medication orders are used in the inpatient or institutional health system setting. Inpatient orders are legal orders that can be used for medications, consultations, laboratory tests, procedures, etc.

There are four types of order. Standing orders are medications given on a regular basis until a patient is discharged or the order is otherwise cancelled. P.R.N. orders are for medications administered only when needed or requested. The order indicates how frequently the medication may be given. Single (One time) Order and stat order.

The following is a listing of commonly used medical orders

Admit orders to the hospital

Admit/transfer to (service:　).

Patient identification：＿＿＿the floor，＿＿＿room, bed (xxx-x)

213

Care teams

Admitting Intern____Pager number____

Admitting Resident____pager number____

Admitting attending____pager number____

Med. rec

Diagnosis:_____

Patient condition

Critical (imminence), unstable, stable, fair, emergent, serious, guarded, not to be released.

Diet orders

Regular diet, liquid (semi-liquid) diet, soft diet, low salt and low fat diet, very low sodium, salt-free diet, low purine diet, low (non)-residue diet, light diet, high caloric diet, high protein (protein-rich) diet, diabetic diet, gestational diabetic, nephritic diet, phosphorus and potassium restricted renal diet, nasal feeding, fasting NPO(nothing by mouth), no eating or drinking, NPO for 5 hours, chylic leak, clear liquid, carbohydrate (carb) controlled, dysphagia, gastric bypass, hyperemesis gravidarum (HG) dry diet.

Activity orders

Bed rest: absolute rest, stay on the bed, bed rest with bathroom privileges, crib and mother's arms, ad lib, no restrictions in the ward.

Nursing orders

Routine: on grade I (II, III), morning (evening) care, bedsore care, mouth (oral) care, accurate input and output values, daily weight, calorie counts, CR (cardiorespiratory) monitor, pulse oximetry, immobilization, or pressed by sand bag.

Parameter: ECG , BP, and SaO_2 monitoring, allergies,

CPT (chest physical therapy), etc.

O$_2$ inhalation NC (2~4L/min via nasal cannula), alcohol sponge bath, cold (hot) compress, wet (hydropathic) compress by MgSO$_4$, change position, gastric lavage with water, bladder irrigation, under water seal drainage of thorax, GI decompression, keep warm, lower temperature by ice-cap, keep bowels open, keep the airway open, retention catheterization, prevent from bedsore, on bedside isolation, raising the head (foot) of the bed, penicillin (procaine, iodine) skin test, intubate and ventilator support, cleaning (retention) enema, soapsuds (saline) enema, intradermal injection, subcutaneous (hypodermic) injection, intramuscular injection(I.M.), intravenous injection(I.V.), intravenous drip(i.v. gtt).

Laboratory test orders

Blood routine tests

Complete blood count (CBC): WBC (white blood count), RBC (red blood count) and PLT (platelet count), Ret (reticulocyte), Hct (hematocrit), MCV (mean corpuscular volume), MCH (mean corpuscular hemoglobin), EC (eosinophic count).

Blood type and screen (T&S), type & cross match blood (T&C) test.

Urinalysis

Uric acid, uric (serum) amylase, urine K$^+$ (Na$^+$), pregnancy test, urine Bence-Jones protein, urinary protein electrophoresis, bacterial count of urine, osmotic pressure assay, 24-hour proteinuria, uric keto-body.

Stool routine examination

Stool ob, stool ova count

215

Coagulation tests

BT (bleeding time), CT (coagulation time), PT (prothrombin time), ACT (activated coagulation time), APTT (kaolin partial thromboplastin time), FIB (fibrinogen), FDP (fibrinogen degradation product), D-dimer fragments assay, capillary resistance test, platelet adhesion and aggregation test, 3P test (plasma, protamine para coagulation test).

Clinical biochemistry

Serum electrolytes(K^+, Na^+, Ca^{2+}, Cl^-, Mg^{2+}), Hcy(homocysteine), Cr and BUN (creatinine and blood urea nitrogen), blood lipid (TG, TC, HDL, LDL), myocardial enzyme (CK, CK-MB, GOT, LDH), Mb (myoglobin), CTn-I, serum iron assay, Vit B_{12} and folic acid assay, ABG (arterial blood gas), renal function and liver function, thyroid function (T_3, T_4, TSH, FT_3 FT_4, TG, TM), LH, FSH, ACTH, GH, determination of calcitonin, 17-KS and 17-OHCS, plasma cortisol assay, aldosterone assay, testosterone and estradiol, FBS or blood glucose, SaO_2 monitor, CO_2CP (carbon dioxide combining power), AFP(alpha-fetoprotein), β_2-M(β_2-microglobulin), plasma viscosity, CSF (cerebrospinal fluid), semen (sputum, vaginal discharge) examination, total protein, albumin/globulin (A/G) ratio, OGTT (oral glucose tolerance test), ANA (antinuclear antibody), anti-ENA antibody, anti-dsDNA, CRP (C-reactive protein), RF(rheumatoid factor), Wilda`s reaction, beta-2 microglobulin tumor marker.

Infection labs

Urine (blood, stool) culture, Pap smear, herpes testing, rubella test, syphilis tests, West Nile virus testing, toxoplasmosis testing, Epstein-Barr virus (EBV) antibody tests, arbovirus testing, viral hepatitis panel, fungal tests.

Radiology / Imaging orders

Ultrasound, ECG (electrocardiogram), EMG(electromyogram), EEG (electroencephalogram), X-ray examination, TTE(transthoracic echo), TEE(transesophageal echo), Doppler echocardiography, fluoroscopy, CT (computerized-tomography), MRI (magnetic resonance imaging), DSA (digital subtractive angiography), contrast enhancement, angiography, coronary angiography, stent, pacemaker implanted operation, Holter (dynamic ECG), treadmill test, bicycle ergometer, TEAP (transesophageal atrial pacing), EP study, barium enema, arterio venography, cholangiography, intravenous (oral) cholecystography, pancreato-cholangiography, selective heptatic arteriography, bronchography, ERCP (endoscopic retrograde cholangio-pancreatography), IVU (intravenous urography), retrograde pyelography, cerebral angiography, vertebral angiography, cisternography, lung functional examination.

Procedure orders

Gastroscopy, endoscopy, sigmoidoscopy, colonoscopy, colonofiberscopy, bronchoscopy, lung aspiration biopsy, catheterization, thoracentesis, abdominocentesis (abdominal puncture), pericardiocentesis, duodenal drainage, liver (renal) biopsy, bone marrow puncture, lumbar puncture, lymph node puncture, joint cavity paracentesis, examination of prostate, CVP (central venous pressure) measure, peripheral venous pressure measure.

（6）医嘱示例 Common Medical Orders Sample

Admit to: Inpatient Service Area;2-12-40

217

Care Team: Maternal and fetal medicine

Admitting Physician: Dr. Yuan Wei

Pager:1561120××××

Attending Physician: Dr. Yang Chen

Pager: 1561156××××

Condition: Good

Allergies: No known drug allergies (NKDA)

Vital Signs: Q 6 h×4, Ward routine, per routine

Activity:　Out of bed/up to chair every 6 hours

Diet: Regular diet

Nursing: per routine, NST tid

Labs:

CBC w/differential　w/ Platelet count

Comprehensive metabolic panel (CMP) / Chem 14

PT or INR/PTT/fibrinogen/TT

Urinalysis - collection method: _____

Urine culture

Blood culture - Collection method: _____

Sets: _____

Type of culture: Bacteria

Sputum culture

Urine hCG

Serum hCG

Thyroid function tests (Specify)

Blood bank:

Type and cross match

Type and screen

For 2 units of packed red blood cells (10~15 ml/kg)

Imaging:

OB ultrasound Urgency

Pre-Op Signed & Held

Total abdominal hysterectomy with xxx MD on 2/28/2019 at 7:30AM

ID	Description	Signed by	When	Reason
249181588	verify informed consent-once (routine)	Xxx MD	02/15/19 1552	RN will Release
249181587	place sequential compression device -knee high, bilateral continuous	Xxx MD	02/15/19 1552	RN will Release
249181588	insert peripheral intravenous-once (routine)	Xxx MD	02/15/19 1552	RN will Release
249184815	maintain intravenous access-continuous	Xxx MD	02/15/19 1552	RN will Release
249184816	sodium chloride 0.9% flush 0.5~20ml-as needed	Xxx MD	02/15/19 1552	RN will Release
249184817	cefazolin (ancef) 2000mg/20ml in sterile water (premix) 2.000mg-once	Xxx MD	02/15/19 1552	RN will Release
249184818	metronidazole(flagyl) 500mg/100ml in sodium chloride (premix) 500mg-once	Xxx MD	02/15/19 1552	RN will Release
249184819	gabapentin(neurontin) capsule 300mg-once	Xxx MD	02/15/19 1552	RN will Release
249184820	acetaminophen (tylenol) tablet 975mg-once	Xxx MD	02/15/19 1552	RN will Release

Pre-Op Signed & Held

Laparoscopic salpingectomy bilateral with xxx MD on 2/28/2019 at 12:30PM

ID	Description	Signed by	When	Reason
243361509	verify informed consent-once (routine)	Xxx MD	01/24/19 1557	RN will Release
243361510	place sequential compression device -knee high, bilateral leg continuous	Xxx MD	01/24/19 1557	RN will Release
243361511	insert peripheral intravenous-once (routine)	Xxx MD	01/24/19 1557	RN will Release
243361512	maintain intravenous access-continuous	Xxx MD	01/24/19 1557	RN will Release
243376476	sodium chloride 0.9% flush 0.5～20ml-as needed	Xxx MD	01/24/19 1557	RN will Release
243376480	sodium chloride 0.9% continuous infusion	Xxx MD	01/24/19 1557	RN will Release
247063792	vital signs-once (routine)	Xxx MD	02/07/19 1707	RN will Release

continue

ID	Description	Signed by	When	Reason
247063793	notify provider of temperature greater than 38.5℃, temperature less than 36℃, systolic blood pressure greater than 180mmHg, systolic blood pressure less than 90mmHg, diastolic blood pressure greater than 100mmH, diastolic blood pressure less than 50mmHg... continuous	Xxx MD	02/07/19 1707	RN will Release
247063794	insert peripheral intravenous-once (Routine)	Xxx MD	02/07/19 1707	RN will Release
247063795	maintain intravenous access-continuous	Xxx MD	02/07/19 1707	RN will Release

Active pre-op orders: Dilation and curettage (D&C)

To start_____ordered

Issuing Time of Medical Orders	Medical Orders	Execution Time of Medical Orders
02/27/19 0636	nursing communication-place OSA sign continuous discontinue comments: place OSA risk sign on bed	02/27/19 0635
02/27/19 0636	OSA precautious continuous discontinue comments: initiate OSA precautious.	02/27/19 0635
02/27/19 0636	insert peripheral intravenous once(routine) discontinue	02/27/19 0635
02/27/19 0636	maintain intravenous access continuous discontinue comments: peripheral intravenous transparent dressing	02/27/19 0635
02/27/19 0636	notify provider temperature greater than 38.5, temperature less than 36℃, systolic blood pressure greater than 180℃, systolic blood pressure less than 90℃, diastolic blood pressure greater than 100 ℃, diastolic blood pressure less than 50℃... continuous discontinue	02/27/19 0635

continue

Issuing Time of Medical Orders	Medical Orders	Execution Time of Medical Orders
02/27/19 0636	POCT glucose stat discontinue	02/27/19 0635
02/27/19 0636	vital signs once (routine) complete discontinue comments: vital signs once upon admission...	02/27/19 0635
02/27/19 0636	insert peripheral intravenous once (routine) discontinue	02/27/19 0635
02/27/19 0636	maintain intravenous access continuous discontinue comments: peripheral intravenous intravenous transparent dress...	02/27/19 0635
02/27/19 0636	place sequential compression device -knee high. bilateral leg continuous discontinue	02/27/19 0635
02/27/19 0636	verify informed consent once (routine) discontinue	02/27/19 0635
02/27/19 0636	sodium chloride 0.9% flush 0.5~20ml as needed discontinue	02/27/19 0635
02/27/19 0636	sodium chloride 0.9% flush 0.5~20ml as needed discontinue	02/27/19 0635

Active PACU Orders

To start _____ ordered

Issuing Time of Medical Orders	Medical Orders	Execution Time of Medical Orders
02/27/19 1015	acetaminophen (tylenol) tablet 1000 mg once discontinue comments: is ok with acetaminophen on it...	02/27/19 0932
02/27/19 0933	pulse oximetry, continuous- phase 1 continuous discontinue	02/27/19 0932
02/27/19 0933	cardiorespiratory monitor - phase 1 continuous discontinue	02/27/19 0932
02/27/19 0933	vital signs - phase 2 per unit routine discontinue	02/27/19 0932
02/27/19 0933	pulse oximetry. continuous - phase 2 continuous discontinue	02/27/19 0932
02/27/19 0933	cardiorespiratory monitor - phase 2 continuous discontinue	02/27/19 0932
02/27/19 0933	notify provider of temperature greater than 38.5℃, temperature less than 36℃, systolic blood pressure greater than 180℃, systolic blood pressure less than 90℃, diastolic blood pressure greater than 100℃, diastolic blood pressure less than 50℃... continuous discontinue	02/27/19 0932

continue

Issuing Time of Medical Orders	Medical Orders	Execution Time of Medical Orders
02/27/19 0933	nursing communication continuous discontinue comments: do not administer narcotics if...	02/27/19 0932
02/27/19 0933	oxygen therapy - continuous discontinue	02/27/19 0932
02/27/19 0933	naloxone (narcan) 0.4mg/ml injection 0.04~0.4mg once as needed discontinue	02/27/19 0932
02/27/19 0933	fentanyl (sublimaze) preservative free injection 50mg once as needed discontinue	02/27/19 0932
02/27/19 0933	ondansetron (zofran) injection 4mg (ondansetron then prochlorperazine progressive panel) once as needed discontinue	02/27/19 0932
02/27/19 0933	prochlorperazine (compazine) injection 10mg (ondansetron then prochlorperazine progressive panel) once as needed discontinue	02/27/19 0932

Admission, transfer, discharge orders: Cesarean section

To start_____ordered

Issuing Time of Medical Orders	Medical Orders	Execution Time of Medical Orders
02/26/19 0946	transfer patient once (routine)	02/26/19 0946
02/26/19 0945	transfer patient once (routine)	02/26/19 0945
02/26/19 0750	assign patient status once (routine)	02/26/19 0750

Active intra-op orders

To start_____ordered

Issuing Time of Medical Orders	Medical Orders	Execution Time of Medical Orders
02/26/19 1000	sodium chloride 0.9% irrigation as needed discontinue	02/26/19 1017
02/26/19 1000	sterile water irrigation as needed discontinue	02/26/19 1019

No phase of care

To start _____ ordered

Issuing Time of Medical Orders	Medical Orders	Execution Time of Medical Orders
02/27/19 1200	acetaminophen (tylenol) tablet 1000mg (acetaminophen or ibuprofen based regimens) every 6 hours scheduled discontinue	02/26/19 1445
02/27/19 1000	oxycodone (roxicodone) tablet 5mg every 4 hours P.R.N. discontinue	02/26/19 1446
02/27/19 0746	vital signs every 4 hours discontinue	02/26/19 1445
02/27/19 0746	ondansetron oot (zofran-odt) disintegrating tablet 4mg (ondansetron I.V. or p.o. panel) every 6 hours P.R.N. discontinue "OR" linked group details	02/26/19 1445
02/27/19 0745	ondansetron (zofran) injection 4mg (ondansetron I.V. or p.o. panel) every 6 hours P.R.N. discontinue "OR" linked group details	02/26/19 1445
02/27/19 0619	foley catheter-discontinue in am once (routine) discontinue	02/27/19 0618
02/27/19 0000	patient may shower with assist continuous discontinue comments: postoperative day 1 after seco....	02/26/19 1445
02/26/19 2100	docusate sodium (colace) capsule 100mg 2 times daily discontinue	02/26/1.9 1445

continue

Issuing Time of Medical Orders	Medical Orders	Execution Time of Medical Orders
02/26/19 1900	ketorolac (toradol) injection 30 mg every 6 hours discontinue	02/26/19 1819
02/26/19 1600	intake and output every 8 hours discontinue comments: till I.V. and/or foley discontinued	02/26/19 1445
02/26/19 1600	breast care every 2 hours discontinue comments: apply ice bags to breasts for...	02/26/19 1445
02/26/19 1530	sodium chloride 0.9% flush 0.5~20ml (maintain I.V. postpartum) every 8 hours scheduled discontinue	2/26/19 1445
02/26/19 1530	oxytocin 30unit/500ml (0.06unit/ml) in sodium chloride 0.9% (premix) solution continuous discontinue	02/26/19 1445
02/26/19 1530	polyethylene glycol (miraiax) packet 17g daily discontinue PNV	02/26/19 1445
02/26/19 1530	with calcium-iron-fa tablet 1 tablet daily discontinue	02/26/19 1445
02/26/19 1446	full code - full CPR continuous discontinue	02/26/19 1445
02/26/19 1446	adult diet regular diet effective now discontinue	02/26/19 1445
02/26/19 1446	activity order strict bed rest until discontinued discontinue comments: for 6 to 8 hours - until alert...	02/26/19 1445
02/26/19 1446	activity order dangle until discontinued discontinue comments: at 6 to 12 hours, chair or amb...	02/26/19 1445

Active pre- op orders -Cesarean section

To start_____ordered

Issuing Time of Medical Orders	Medical Orders	Execution Time of Medical Orders
02/26/19 1446	activity order dangle until discontinued discontinue comments: at 6 to 12 hours, chair or amb...	02/26/19 1445
02/26/19 1446	notify provider temperature greater than 38℃, systolic blood pressure greater than 140℃, systolic blood pressure less than 90mmHg, diastolic blood pressure greater than 90mmHg, diastolic blood pressure less than 60mmHg, heart rate greater than 120 beats per minute. He... Continuous Discontinue	02/26/19 1445
02/26/19 1446	nursing communication-apply abdominal binder once (routine) complete discontinue	02/26/19 1445
02/26/19 1446	breast pump once (routine) complete discontinue comments: if breast feeding	02/26/19 1445
02/26/19 1446	place sequential compression device-(exclusion for DVT drug prophylaxis but with SCO order) continuous discontinue "and" linked group details	02/26/19 1445

continue

Issuing Time of Medical Orders		Medical Orders	Execution Time of Medical Orders
02/26/19	1446	maintain I.V. access (maintain I.V. postpartum) continuous discontinue comments: peripheral I.V. transparent dress...	02/26/19 1445
02/26/19	1446	apply lanolin ointment continuous discontinue comments: apply as needed to sore/irritate...	02/26/19 1445
02/26/19	1446	apply tucks pad continuous discontinue comments: apply tucks pad as needed for...	02/26/19 1445
02/26/19	1446	patient does not meet requirements for rbogam once (routine) complete discontinue comments: rhogam is not needed, patient ...	02/26/19 1445
02/26/19	1446	consult to lactation once (routine) complete discontinue provider: (not yet assigned)	02/26/19 1445
02/26/19	1446	activity order strict bed rest until discontinued discontinue comments: strict bedrest until dc of spi...	02/26/19 1445
02/26/19	1446	elevate hob until discontinued discontinue comments: elevate hob 30 degrees minimum...	02/26/19 1445
02/26/19	1446	vital signs continuous discontinue comments: include pain score, and POSS	02/26/19 1445

continue

Issuing Time of Medical Orders	Medical Orders	Execution Time of Medical Orders
02/26/19 1446	continuous pulse oximetry continuous discontinue	02/26/19 1445
02/26/19 1446	notify provider temperature greater than 38.5℃, temperature less than 36℃, systolic blood pressure greater than 160mmHg, systolic blood pressure less than 90mmHg diastolic blood pressure greater than 90mmHg, diastolic blood pressure less than 50mmHg continuous discontinue	02/26/19 1445
02/26/19 1446	notify provider notify anesthesia for epidural or spinal pain management issues. continuous discontinue comments: notify anesthesia for epidural...	02/26/19 1445
02/26/19 1446	notify provider notify anesthesia for decreased sensory level above the nipple line. continuous discontinue comments: notify anesthesia for decrease...	02/26/19 1445

231

continue

Issuing Time of Medical Orders		Medical Orders	Execution Time of Medical Orders
02/26/19	1446	notify provider notify anesthesia for severe back pain. continuous discontinue comments: notify anesthesia for severe …	02/26/19 1445
02/26/19	1446	notify provider notify anesthesia for neurological changes or deterioration. continuous discontinue comments: notify anesthesia for neurology…	02/26/19 1445
02/26/19	1446	notify provider notify anesthesia for nausea/vomiting… fetal distress, extreme anxiety, or difficulty breathing. continuous discontinue comments. notify anesthesia for nausea/v…	02/26/19 1445
02/26/19	1446	no antiplatelet (except aspirin) continuous discontinue comments: contact anesthesia prior to or…	02/26/19 1445
02/26/19	1446	no anticoagulants continuous discontinue comments: contact anesthesia prior to or...	02/26/19 1445
02/26/19	1446	nursing communication: all opioid management per anesthesia for 24 hours continuous discontinue comments: all opioid management per anesthesia team	02/26/19 1445
02/26/19	1446	oxygen therapy continuous discontinue comments: place patient on non-rebreathe...	02/26/19 1445

continue

Issuing Time of Medical Orders		Medical Orders	Execution Time of Medical Orders
02/26/19	1445	naloxone (narcan) 0.4mg/ml injection 0.04~0.4mg once as needed discontinue	02/26/19 1445
02/26/19	1445	sodium chloride 0.9% flush 0.5~20ml (maintain I.V. postpartum) as needed discontinue	02/26/19 1445
02/26/19	1445	simethicone (mylicon) chewable tablet 80mg 4 times daily P.R.N. (after meals, bedtime) Discontinue	02/26/19 1445
02/26/19	1445	hydrocortisone (anusol-hc) 2.5% rectal cream 3 times daily P.R.N discontinue	02/26/19 1445
02/26/19	1418	oxycodone (roxicodone) tablet 5mg (p.o. opioids) every 4 hours P.R.N discontinue	02/26/19 1418
02/26/19	1308	ondansetron (zofran) injection 4mg every 6 hours P.R.N discontinue us ob limited once (routine) discontinue	02/26/19 1308
02/26/19	0751	straight catheterize as needed discontinue comments: if no void in 6 hours, straight catheter	02/26/19 0750

233

Admission, Transfer. Discharge Orders-delivery

To start   ordered

Issuing Time of Medical Orders		Medical Orders	Execution Time of Medical Orders	
02/27/19	0840	transfer patient once (routine)	02/27/19	0839
02/27/19	0238	transfer patient once (routine)	02/27/19	0239
02/26/19	1802	assign patient status once (routine)	02/26/19	1807

Active Pre-op Orders

To start   ordered

Issuing Time of Medical Orders		Medical Orders	Execution Time of Medical Orders	
02/26/19	1812	CBC without differential STAT	02/26/19	1812
02/26/19	1811	calcium gluconate 100mg/ml (10%) injection 1g (magnesium sulfate for pre-eclampsia) once as needed discontinue	02/26/19	1812

No Phase of Care
To start

ordered

Issuing Time of Medical Orders	Medical Orders	Execution Time of Medical Orders
02/28/19 0235	magnesium sulfate in lactated Ringer's 25g/300ml infusion (premix) (magnesium sulfate for pre-eclampsia) continuous discontinue	02/27/19 1009
02/28/19 0037	ondansetron odt (zofran-odt) disintegrating tablet 4mg (ondansetron I.V. or p.o. panel) every 6 hours P.R.N. discontinue "of" linked group details	02/27/19 0839
02/28/19 0037	ondansetron (zofran) injection 4mg (ondansetron I.V. or p.o. panel) Every 6 hours P.R.N discontinue"or" linked group details	02/27/19 0839
02/27/19 2100	enoxaparin (lovenox) syringe 40mg daily (for enoxaparin) discontinue	02/27/19 0839

continue

Issuing Time of Medical Orders	Medical Orders	Execution Time of Medical Orders
02/27/19 1300	CBC with auto differential timed draw discontinue	02/27/19 1042
02/27/19 1300	comprehensive metabolic panel once (routine) discontinue	02/27/19 1042
02/27/19 1300	fibrinogen once (routine) discontinue	02/27/19 1042
02/27/19 1300	protime-INR once (routine) discontinue	02/27/19 1042
02/27/19 1300	APTT once (routine) discontinue	02/27/19 1042
02/27/19 1200	breast care every 4 hours discontinue comments: apply ice bags to breasts for...	02/27/19 0839
02/27/19 1045	dextrose 5% and lactated ringer's infusion continuous discontinue	02/27/19 1008
02/27/19 0945	nifedipine (procardia xl/adalat cc) extended release tablet 30mg daily discontinue	02/27/19 0907

continue

Issuing Time of Medical Orders	Medical Orders	Execution Time of Medical Orders
02/27/19 0915	Rho(D) immune globulin (hyperrho S/D RhoGAM) injection 300mg once discontinue	02/27/19 0839
02/27/19 0915	oxytocin 30 unit/500ml (0.06unit/ml) in sodium chloride 0.9% (premix) solution continuous discontinue	02/27/19 0839
02/27/19 0915	docusate sodium (colace) capsule 100mg 2 times daily discontinue	02/27/19 0839
02/27/19 0915	polyethylene glycol (miralax) packet 17g daily discontinue	02/27/19 0839
02/27/19 0915	PNV with calcium-iron-FA tablet 1 tablet daily discontinue	02/27/19 0839
02/27/19 0840	full code - full cpr continuous discontinue	02/27/19 0839
02/27/19 0840	activity order up with assist until discontinued discontinue comments: until sensation returns from e...	02/27/19 0839
02/27/19 0840	activity order up ad lib until discontinued discontinue comments: once epidural wears off	02/27/19 0839

To start

ordered

Issuing Time of Medical Orders	Medical Orders	Execution Time of Medical Orders
02/27/19 0840	full code - full CPR continuous discontinue	02/27/19 0839
02/27/19 0840	activity order up with assist until discontinued discontinue comments: until sensation returns from ...	02/27/19 0839
02/27/19 0840	activity order up ad lib until discontinued discontinue comments: once epidural wears off	02/27/19 0839
02/27/19 0840	patient may shower daily discontinue	02/27/19 0839
02/27/19 0840	vital signs continuous discontinue comments: vitals every 15 minutes for 2 ...	02/27/19 0839
02/27/19 0840	notify provider temperature greater than 38°C, systolic blood pressure greater than 140mmHg, systolic blood pressure less than 90mmHg, diastolic blood pressure greater than 90mmHg, diastolic blood pressure less than 60mmHg, heart rate greater than 120beats per minute, continuous discontinue	02/27/19 0839
02/27/19 0840	check fundus continuous discontinue	02/27/19 0839

continue

Issuing Time of Medical Orders	Medical Orders	Execution Time of Medical Orders
02/27/19 0840	nursing communication - check lochia continuous discontinue	02/27/19 0839
02/27/19 0840	breast pump once (routine) complete discontinue comments: if breastfeeding	02/27/19 0839
02/27/19 0840	nursing communication - discontinue I.V. once (routine) complete discontinue comments: remove I.V. 12 hours postpartum ...	02/27/19 0839
02/27/19 0840	fundal massage - vigorously for minimum of 15 seconds. every 15min discontinue	02/27/19 0839
02/27/19 0840	vital signs - every 5 minutes every 5 min discontinue	02/27/19 0839
02/27/19 0840	fundal massage - vigorously for minimum of 15 seconds. every 15 minutes discontinue	02/27/19 0839
02/27/19 0840	apply lanolin ointment continuous discontinue comments: apply as needed to sore/irrita...	02/27/19 0839
02/27/19 0840	apply tucks pad continuous discontinue comments: apply tucks pad as needed for ...	02/27/19 0839

continue

Issuing Time of Medical Orders	Medical Orders	Execution Time of Medical Orders
02/27/19 0840	consult to lactation once (routine) complete discontinue provider: (not yet assigned)	02/27/19 0839
02/27/19 0840	patient does not meet requirements for rhogam once (routine) complete discontinue comments: rhogam is not needed, patient...??	02/27/19 0839
02/27/19 0839	measles-mumps-rubeila (MMR) 1000~12500 TCID 50/0.5ml vaccine 0.5ml during hospitalization discontinue	02/27/19 0839
02/27/19 0839	acetaminophen (tylenol) tablet 650mg (acetaminophen or ibuprofen based regimens) every 4 hours P.R.N. discontinue	02/27/19 0839
02/27/19 0839	benzocaine-menthol! (dermoplast) 20%~0.5% topical spray 1 spray as needed discontinue	02/27/19 0839
02/27/19 0839	hydrocortisone (anusol-hc) 2.5% rectal cream 3 times daily P.R.N. discontinue	02/27/19 0839
02/27/19 0703	NPO diet effective now discontinue	02/27/19 0702

continue

Issuing Time of Medical Orders	Medical Orders	Execution Time of Medical Orders
02/27/19 0400	oxytocin 30unit/500ml (0.06 unit/ml) in sodium chloride 0.9% (premix) solution continuous	02/27/19 0323
02/27/19 0310	loperamide (imodium) capsule 2mg 4 times daily P.R.N. discontinue	02/27/19 0311
02/27/19 1812	fluid restriction - I.V. fluids continuous discontinue	02/27/19 1812
02/27/19 1812	seizure precautions continuous discontinue	02/27/19 1812
02/27/19 1811	calcium gluconate 100 mg/ml (10%) injection 1 g (magnesium sulfate for pre-eclampsia) once as needed discontinue	02/27/19 1812
Unscheduled	straight catheterize as needed discontinue comments: if no void in 6 hours, catheterization	02/27/19 0839
Unscheduled	weigh blood loss every 5～15 minutes as needed discontinue	02/27/19 0839
Unscheduled	assess - ail vaginal walls, cervix, uterine cavity, and rule out retained poc, laceration or hematoma as needed discontinue	02/27/19 0839

5. 病例报告写作 Writing a Case Report

A medical case report is an article that describes a patient's diagnosis and treatment procedure. Most of the cases chosen for writing reports are characterized by unusual diagnoses or with complications during hospitalization. A medical case report should be submitted in a specific formation in accordance to the requirements of peer-reviewed journals. To write a medical case report, you should first obtain the proper consent to write and publish the report, and then collect information about the patient. A good case report should keep the readers interested in the situation and provide enough information for the readers to understand the problem.

（1）病例报告写作原则 Principles of Writing a Case Report

You have five steps to be done when writing a case report.

Step 1. Select a case

Pay attention to patients who have rare or unusual illnesses, and keep eyes open on the treatment plans that have an unexpected positive or negative outcome. Talk with senior physicians about patients whose illnesses would make an interesting case study report.

The meaningful case should meet at least one of the following criteria:

1) Presentations, diagnoses and/or management of new and emerging diseases.

2) Unexpected or unusual presentations of a disease.

3) New associations or variations in disease processes.

4) Unreported or unusual side effects or adverse actions involving medications.

5) An unexpected event in the course of observing or treating a patient.

6) New findings revealed pathogenesis of a disease or an adverse effect.

Step 2. Search and review the literature

- Search and review the literature on the diagnosis or treatment that will be the focus of your case report. This information will be a significant part of your paper once you begin writing.

Step 3. Collect patient information and obtain consent

- Medical and publication ethics require that the patient who you will report must provide written consent before you submit your report.

- Collect the patient's demographic information (age, medical history, medication use, current and past diagnoses, etc.). Provide detailed information about the patient so that your audience will be well informed about the case.

- Get copies of the patient's labs, X-rays or any clinical photographs.

Step 4. Write the manuscript

- Follow the standard format for case report, including abstract, introduction, case presentation, discussion, conclusion and references. Pay attention to the writer's guidelines for the publication provided by the journal you choose.

243

Step 5. Submit your case report to an academic journal

Before submitting the manuscript, you should tell the editor and reviewer what your case adds to the field of medicine. In your cover letter, please consider the following: Whether it is the first report of this kind of disease in the literature? Will it significantly advance our understanding of a particular disease etiology or drug mechanism?

（2）病例报告文字写作内容 Preparation of Manuscript of Case Reports

Firstly, you should select a proper professional journal to submit your report. This journal should cover the area of your scientific research. Then read the "Instruction to the Author" section carefully. Each journal has its unique format. In the following part, we will introduce the usual format of most journals. Manuscripts for case reports submitted to medical journals should be divided into the following sections (in the following order):

- Title page
- Abstract
- Keywords
- Introduction
- Case presentations
- Discussion
- Conclusions
- Consent
- Competing interests
- Authors' contributions

- Acknowledgements
- References

Title page

The first page of the manuscript should be a detailed title page, including the title of the article, full names of author(s), affiliation(s) and address(es), corresponding author name and contact information, word count of the manuscript. The title of the article should be concise and informative.

Title example 1:

Coronary artery dissection, traumatic liver and spleen injury after cardiopulmonary resuscitation: A case report.

Title example 2:

Anterior medial meniscal root avulsions due to malposition of the tibial tunnel during anterior cruciate ligament reconstruction: Two case reports.

Or, if the case reports details several patients.

Title example 3:

Clinico radiological characteristics of patients with differentiated thyroid carcinoma and renal metastasis: Case series with follow up.

Some journals permit the author to recommend one or two reviewers in the related scientific area if the disease or medical problem is too rare or too complex for most reviewers. The recommended reviewers should not be in the authors' list. It is better not to recommend reviewers from the same institute as the authors. For most of the journals, it is authors' authority to refuse some reviewers to the editorial board. In the submission process, the author should list the names and institutions of the refused reviewers.

Abstract

This part should be in the second page of the manuscript. The abstract is normally 200 to 350 words, and words account must less than the journal's limitation. Abbreviations or references should not exist in the abstract. The abstract includes three sections and should emphasize the meaning of adding this case report into clinical literature:

- Introduction

Introduction about the importance of reporting this case. This includes information on whether this kind of cases is first reported in the literature.

- Case presentation

Describe the details of the case briefly, including the age, sex and ethnic background.

- Conclusion

Briefly conclude what can be learned from this case and its clinical impact. Talk about whether it is the case firstly reported in the specialized area and what effects it will have on medicine development and advancing our knowledge about the etiology and therapy of a particular disease.

Keywords

The number of the key words is not restricted, usually three to six. The more important the keyword is, the more prior position it should be put. Key words may present research area of the case, and help Editorial board to invite reviewers in relevant areas.

Introduction

Introduction should supply the case background

information, containing the disorder, usual presentation, disease progression, and if it is a new disease. A brief literature review should also be included in the introduction.

Case presentations

In this section, all details related to the case should be present, including the patient's demographic information (patient's personal information should be protected), symptoms, signs, medical history, lab tests and therapy. A case series should contain details of all patients.

Discussion

Discussion is an optional section, additional comments in this part can provide relevant information not included in the case presentation, and explanation of specific treatment decisions can also be included in discussion.

Conclusions

State the main conclusion and explain its importance in advancing the knowledge of this specialized area from the medical perspective. Talk about if it is an original case report of a particular area and its influence in the medicine progression. Please mention that how this case significantly helps doctors figure out the etiology, presentation, progression and treatment of a particular disease.

Consent

This section is compulsory. Informed consent is required before manuscripts are peer-reviewed, and it shows that patients has given their informed consent for the case report publishment. Following words are recommended in consent section: "Written informed consent was obtained from the patient for publication of this case report and accompanying images. A copy of the written consent is available for review by the Editor-in-Chief of this journal".

Competing interests

Authors are required to write competing interests declaration. All declared competing interests should be listed at the end of published articles. If there is no competing interests declared, it will be written "The author(s) declare that they have no competing interests" at the end.

Authors' contributions

Contributions of each author to the manuscript should be specified in this section to give appropriate credit to individual author. We recommend the following kinds of formats (initials are used to refer to each author's contribution): ××× initiated the idea and design the scientific research or medical case. ××× finished follow-up of patients. ××× analyzed and interpreted the patient data. ××× supervised and organized the course of the project and the manuscript. ××× is the major contributor in manuscript writing up. All authors read and approved the final manuscript.

Acknowledgements

Indicate the source(s) of research fund for each author, and for the manuscript preparation. Contributors who do not meet the criteria for authorship can be listed in this section, such as persons who provided technical help, data acquisition and interpretation help, or revised the draft manuscript critically.

References

The relevant case reports have been published must

be searched and cited. Different journals have different requirements for reference formats.

Usually use following style:

Authors

Title of the article

Journal

Published year

Volume (issue)

Page number

Example 1 (all authors):

WAY, K. L., HACKETT, D. A., BAKER, M. K. & JOHNSON, N. A. The effect of regular exercise on insulin sensitivity in type 2 diabetes mellitus: A systematic review and meta-analysis. Diabetes & metabolism journal, 2016, 40: 253-271.

Example 2 (the first three authors):

WAY K. L., HACKETT D. A., BAKER M. K et al. The effect of regular exercise on insulin sensitivity in type 2 diabetes mellitus: A systematic review and meta-analysis. Diabetes & metabolism journal, 2016, 40: 253-271.

Example 3 (article within a journal supplement):

FRUMIN AM. Functional asplenia: Demonstration of splenic activity by bone marrow scan. Blood, 1979,59 (Suppl) 1:26-32.

Example 4 (books):

JUNBO GE, YONGJIAN XU. Internal medicine [M]. The eighth edition. Beijing: People's Medical Publishing House, 2014.

Example 5 (clinical trial registration record):

DAVIES SJ. (2019): Changing doctors' behavior in

the treatment of low blood pressure. Current Controlled Trials. http://www.isrctn.com/ISRCTN17085700

Example 6 (article in electronic format):

KIM. ER stress drives lipogenesis and steatohepatitis via caspase-2 activation of S1P. Cell (2018), https://doi.org/10.1016/j.cell.2018.08.020

（3）图片 Preparing Illustrations and Figures

Follow the "Instruction for Authors" on the official websites of journals. According to specific instructions of each journal, some can only allow no more than ten figures in each case report to be published. Explain why you need to publish extra figures in your covering letter, if you have more than ten figures and feel that all the figures are essential to the understanding of the case report. Authors are responsible to label all figures and tables sequentially and include all relevant supporting data with each article. Case reports with video/movie images are more favored by some journals.

Illustrations of corresponding figure should not be embedded in the text file, but provided as separate files, and should fit on a single page in portrait format. If a figure consists of separate parts, author should make sure a single composite illustration file with all parts of the figure is submitted. Some journals do not make an extra charge for color figures.

Authors should spare no efforts to help preserve the anonymity of the patients. First, any identifiable features of the participants, including birthmarks and tattoos, should be removed or concealed. Second, please take extra care with images of the head and face, ensuring that only the relevant features are shown. Publication of facial images will be subject to chief editor's approval.

Figure legends

Legends and figures are separate parts. Therefore, figure legends should be included in the main manuscript text file at the end of the document or placed as the journal required. For each figure, the following information should be provided: Figure number (in sequence, using Arabic numerals, i.e. Figure 1, 2, 3 etc), short title of figure, detailed legend.

The exact location of the image on the patient, the type of image (e.g. micrograph/X-ray), and time in relation to progression (e.g. one week after surgery) should be briefly described in an appropriate legend. Abbreviations should not be used unless they are expanded (except for common ones such as antibodies).

It should be noted that the author(s) are responsible to obtain permission from the copyright holder to reproduce figures or tables that have previously been published elsewhere.

（4）表格 Preparing Tables

Please note that the author(s) should number and cite each table in sequence using arabic numerals (i.e. Table 1, 2, 3 etc.). A summary title (above the table) should be given to the whole table, which is followed by detailed but concise legends. Tables should always be cited in the manuscript in consecutive numerical order.

The borders of each table cell display as black lines so that columns and rows of data can be visibly distinct. Commas should not be used to indicate numerical values.

Color and shading should be avoided; important parts of the table can be highlighted with symbols or in bold format, the meaning of which should then be explained in the corresponding table legend. Tables should not be embedded as figures or spreadsheet files.

Large datasets or tables that are too wide for a landscape page can be uploaded separately additional files. Additional files will not be displayed in the final, laid-out PDF of the article, but as a link listed in the text (supplied by the author). These additional files containing tabular data can be uploaded as an Excel spreadsheet (.xls) or comma separated values (.csv) as the journal requires. As with all files, standard file extensions should be used.

（5）其他材料 Preparing Additional Files

Usually, datasets, tables, movies, or other information of case reports are recommended to be uploaded as additional files by the journals, which also have high priority for publication. Additional files will be published along with the article as a link provided by the author. Please note that each journal requires a maximum file size for additional files.

The author(s) should confirm that all files are virus-scanned on submission so that they can be safely downloaded from the final published article provided by the author(s).

Additional files can be in any format according to the requirements of the journal. Please confirm that certain supported file formats can be well recognized by the users and displayed in the browser. Most movie formats, mini-websites prepared according to the guidelines, chemical structure files (MOL, PDB), geographic data files (KML) will be appropriate and easy to open. If the author plans to provide additional materials, please list the following information in a separate section of the manuscript:

- File name (e.g. additional file 1)
- File format with a correct file extension, for example, .pdf, .xls, .txt, .pptx (including name and a URL of an appropriate viewer if unusual format is used)
- Title of data
- Description of data

The author should name the additional files with standard names as "Additional file 1" and so on, and explicitly reference their name in the appropriate sections of the article, e.g. "an additional video file shows this in more details [see additional file 1]".

Style and language

Submitted manuscripts should be written in standard scientific English and which are poorly written will be returned to authors for language revision prior to peers' review. It is highly suggested that all scientific articles should be written clearly and concisely, and be checked by all other colleagues who participated in the research before submission. Non-native English speakers may choose to have their articles edited by a copy editing service.

Please go through your article thoroughly and correct all misused words, spelling errors, missing references or incomplete citation information before submission. Manuscript with too many languages and editing mistakes can result in direct rejection or "re-review" after revision.

Abbreviations

Abbreviations should be defined when first used and

a list of abbreviations should be provided by the author following or in the front of the main manuscript text. It is recommended that abbreviations should be avoided as much as possible.

Units

Author(s) are supposed to use international units throughout the manuscript (liter and molar are permitted).

Case overview

As part of the submission process, you will take a few minutes to answer a series of questions by the editorial board. The following is an outline of the case overview content. It is not prerequisite for authors to prepare this section prior to submission.

Patient details

- Age
- Sex
- Country of residence
- Clinical details
- Reasons for case presentation
- Primary diagnosis
- Secondary diagnosis (if applicable)
- Investigations carried out before diagnosis
- Pharmaceutical preparations
- Geographical location of this report

第四章 英文论文写作
Chapter 4. English Thesis Writing

1. SCI 及影响因子简介 Brief Introduction of SCI and IF

如何进行学术演讲

SCI is the English abbreviation of the American Scientific Citation Index, which is all known as: Science Citation Index, officially launched in 1964. It is based on the idea of citation proposed by the modern intelligence school Engene Garfield in 1953. The Science Citation Index (SCI) is an index originally produced by the Institute for Scientific Information (ISI) and created by the Institute for Scientific Information (ISI) in Philadelphia, USA. SCI, EI (Engineering Index), and ISTP (Index to Scientific &Technical Proceedings) are the world's three major scientific literature retrieval systems. SCI is published by ISI for Scientific, the American Science Intelligence, and is now a bimonthly magazine. The expanded version (SCI expanded) covers more than 8,500 notable and significant journals, across 150 disciplines, from 1 900 to the present. In addition to publishing SCI, ISI also has an online database SCTSEARCH. ISTP is also published by it. SCI is divided into printed version, CD version and online board and other carriers. The Printed and CD editions select 3 300 SCI-tech journals from tens of thousands of journals around the world, covering more than 100 areas of basic science. Annual coverage includes the latest 600,000 articles, involving 9 million citations.

SCI is an international search publication that includes natural science, biology, medicine, agriculture, technology and behavioral science, with a major focus on basic science. The publications are selected from 94 categories, more than 40 countries and a variety of languages. SCI also included a certain number of Chinese publications.

The selection process of periodicals is prudent. It takes the combined methods of citation data analysis and peer evaluation, with the full consideration of the academic value. The collection of more than 3 400 selected journals covers most important international academic journals. As a result, SCI has become an internationally recognized representative tool for reflecting the level of scientific research. Furthermore, the number of SCI papers is regarded as representative of one country's scientific and technological capabilities. As the focus of competition, SCI retrieval system has always been the center of academia and the source of literature statistics worldwide.

This database allows researchers to identify particular earlier articles that later articles have cited, or the articles of any particular author. According to the survey of relevant departments, there are three main aspects of SCI selection: editing quality, citation indicators and expert review, among which citation indicators are the most objective. The SCI system uses its unique citation method and comprehensive scientific data to count quantitative indicators such as impact factors, citation frequency, and real-time index of a certain journal, and then rank journals and papers according to these indicators. The high cited frequency of an article indicates a huge impact in its field and a relatively high academic level. These advantages of SCI are of great help to scientific and technological workers in accessing the latest literature, tracking international academic frontiers, scientific research projects and timely understanding of international developments in specific subjects.

The IF of an academic journal is a measure reflecting the yearly average number of citations to recently published articles. The IF was devised by Eugene Garfield, the founder of the American Institute for Scientific Information, and was used to compare different journals in a certain field.

Referring to the citation frequency of an article in a journal in a particular year or period, IF is an important indicator of the influence of academic journals. In any year, the journal's IF is the number of articles cited in the journal received in the year, divided by the total number of articles published in the journal in the previous two years:

$$IF_y = \frac{Citations_{y-1} + Citations_{y-2}}{Publications_{y-1} + Publications_{y-2}}$$

New journals, which are indexed from their first published issue, will receive an IF after two years of indexing.

2. 医学论文的格式和内容 English Thesis Format and Contents

All scientific papers have the same general format. They are divided into distinct sections and each section contains a specific type of information. It is mainly divided into following parts:

- Title page
- Abstract, and Key words
- Introduction
- Materials and methods
- Results
- Discussion
- Acknowledgments
- Reference
- Graphics and Tables
- Figure legends

Scientific papers often are organized in this way:

Tips1. Title pages

The title page should include:

- The name(s) of the author(s)
- A concise and informative title
- The affiliation(s) and address(es) of the author(s)
- The e-mail address, and telephone number(s) of the corresponding author

The most important part is title, because it is the first part that an editors/reviewers/reader will see. It must present the subject and what aspect of the subject was studied. A good title gives a reasonably complete description of the study that was conducted, and sometimes even foreshadow the findings. Included in a title are the species studied, the kinds of experiments performed, and perhaps a brief indication of the results obtained.

Tips 2. Abstract, and Key words

Abstract: The second page of the scientific paper begins with an abstract, which is the summary of paper and explains the objective of the study, the primary results, the main conclusions. Abstracts are often included in article databases, and are usually free to a large audience. Thus, they may be the most widely read portions of scientific papers. This is a short, all-encompassing section that summarizes what you discussed in the rest of this article and should be written to the end after you know what you said. And must not exceed 250～300 words.

Key words: Provide 4 to 6 keywords which can be used for indexing purposes. The most important keywords should be placed in the prior position.

Tips 3. Introduction

The introduction must provide theoretical background to understand why the work is important, states the research question, and poses a hypothesis to be tested. A well-written "introduction" includes a clear statement of the problem or question to be solved in the experiment, the hypothesis that you tested in the study, why this is an important question to be /or why you found this to be a particularly interesting question, an objective of the research, and how the research helps to fill gaps in our knowledge. In this topic, you can use references to explain.

Tips 4. Materials and methods

The materials and methods describe both specific techniques and the overall experimental reagent used by the authors. It must contain sufficient information. Careful writing of this section is important so that experimental procedures can be reproduced.

Tips 5. Results

The "Results" section presents in words the major

results of the paper. Your data should be presented in detail with diagrams, tables, graphs and text description. However, do not present the same data in different types. Strive for clarity, the results should be clear and pellucid. You should not discuss the interpretation of your data, this should be done in the next section.

Tips 6. Discussion

The discussion follows the results section and should interpret your results in detail, speculating on trends, possible causes, and conclusions. Do not simply reiterate data in the Results. You should state what conclusions can be drawn from the results, put your results in the context of the hypotheses and other material in the introduction, point out where your data fits in to the big picture, compare your results with those of other researches and cite literature to verify the progressiveness and innovation of the results or comparisons, indicate problems in your research, and how to avoid them in the future, try to explain why results might be inconsistent with the predictions you made and interpret unexpected results, draw your major conclusions as clearly as possible!

Tips 7. Acknowledgments

The acknowledgments should tell readers about the contribution of people or institutions (other than the authors) to this work, and the sources of funds that provided financial support for the study.

Tips 8. References

The list of references should only include works that are cited in the text and that have been published or accepted for publication. Personal communications and unpublished works should only be mentioned in the text. The specific reference format should refer to each magazine's own requirements.

Tips 9. Graphics and Tables

This part is not strictly writing, but it is a demonstration of the results of the article and an important part of the article. Good graphics can convey the resulting information to the reader without a lot of text interpretation.

Tips 10. Figure legends

Figure legend is an explanation of the Graphics. It should be comprehensive and easy to understand. Should be placed at the end of the text rather than beside the graphics, each figure should provide a short legend.

In medical research work, SCI must be published, and it must be the clinical cases and research that it has accumulated over the years. In the case of ensuring innovation and originality, but what kind of articles meet the requirements of SCI journals?

1) Original content: The originality of the SCI paper is the most basic. Although the SCI journal did not ask the author to be original, the original individual felt that it was necessary to publish a paper. Recently, there are many SCI paper publishing companies that do not have their own editors. They rely on the process of publishing SCI papers to swindle. Most of the contents written by them are plagiarized. Once such articles are discovered, the consequences are very serious.

2) Clear and organized: If the article's organization is unclear, it will confuse the reviewer, which wastes an innovative idea. When writing the introduction section, such as writing the role of vitamin D_3 in the prevention of esophageal cancer, the following ideas are written: First,

the definition of esophageal cancer, the incidence rate, has brought great harm to human health. Therefore, we investigated the role of plasma vitamin D_3 levels in the prevention of esophageal cancer. This is very random, and it does not reflect why it is to check the level of vitamin D_3 in plasma, rather than the role of its main body metabolite level in the prevention of esophageal cancer.

3) Novel and innovation: No SCI journals will include articles that are not innovative, which is not conducive to the long-term publication of SCI journals, which is obviously different from some low-quality journals in China. A lot of magazines, whose income is funded by sponsors, not district fee.

4) The clear purpose: The purpose of your SCI papers must be clear. If others can't see which aspects of your paper are mainly researched, then do you think your papers will be included in SCI journals?

5) The reliable method: The methodology section can be simple, but it must be repeatable.

6) The verified results: This is not much to say. The essence of the publication of SCI papers is here.

7) Scientific research significance: The discussion of SCI papers does not require the author to further elaborate on the results. A good discussion can highlight the scientific significance of the entire article.

3. 论著论文撰写原则及示例 Principles and Examples of Articles

According to the sources of data, papers are usually divided into two categories: Original papers and edited papers.

Original paper is the summarize of survey research, experimental research, clinical research. It states the first-hand information (also called direct data). It covers extensive contents, including the scientific summarize of the progress on new theory or new technology applied to the practical uses and indirect innovations in medical theory and new scientific research achievements (experimental research, clinical observation, investigation report, case report and case discussion). The original paper is not only an important symbol of the scientific research level, but also the main carrier of scientific hypotheses and viewpoints put forward by researchers.

The main content of edited papers are from the published data and belongs to the third literature, which is based on indirect data. In combination with some personal research data and experience of the author, the scattered, unsystematic, repetitive and even contradictory data from various sources are orchestrated by the author's personal views, so that the readers can know about the latest development in a certain subject or topic in a short time.

Medical papers can promote healthy care, which explores diseases, pathologies, pharmaceutical agents, or new medical technologies. Therefore, the kind of papers can be published as long as they are beneficial to people's healthy, and there are four common types of papers, namely medical theory, case reports, case sequences and medical reviews.

（1）Medical Literature

Generally, medical literatures are divided into

basic and clinical papers, most of the publishing papers are basic article, which belongs to prospective studies. Popular speaking, we make assumptions that the line of thinking and then prove the line of thinking through the conclusion of the experiment, there may be two outcomes, that is positive (conform to ideas) or negative (don't conform to ideas), It's wrong point that the negative result can't be published on the SCI. In fact, the negative results can also published. And one can imagine that the negative results tell us that train of thought can't come out the results, which is also a contribution to international research.

Clinical articles are relatively rare, because most clinicians are busy and don't have free time, and few doctors will devote themselves to clinical research and writing. As for the format and word count requirements of articles, they are generally about 3 500 to 5 000 words, and 20 to 35 references (the best english articles that are published in SCI journals to improve the level of articles).

（2）Case Report

Many clinicians like to publish a case report. They think it is easier to publish a case report than clinical articles. The requirements of the case report are 800 to 1 500 words and 8 to 10 references. Moreover, SCI journals accept case reports, which need to meet one of the following three standards.

1) The case report must be the first case report.

2) The case report must be rare or unique.

3) Is the case report can prove the hypothesis or theory of an expert.

Of course, SCI case reports should meet five standards in writing, all of them that are indispensable.

1) Case reports include the symptoms of the patient who comes into the department.

2) Case reports include the methods of assessment, which are used to detect the disease by the doctors.

3) Case reports include the methods of treatment.

4) Case reports include the result of treatment.

5) Case reports include the follow-up, the situation about the patient discharged and three months after discharging.

（3）Case Sequence

Case sequence is a report including more than three cases, which involve a meta-analysis that is the most difficult analysis in biostatistics.

Significantly, SCI reviews are different from the ones which are published in doctoral or master's theses. The SCI reviews are not published by ordinary people, those are published by people who have a very high status in the medical field and are invited articles by the journal. For example, the journal will send a letter to the authoritative hematology department in the world to invite one professor to summarize the development of the hematology field this year or make an expectation for the future development.

The original article is a type of writing to summarize the research results. Medical treatises include experimental studies, clinical observations (drugs and clinical medicine, manipulation and clinical medicine, diagnostic techniques and clinical medicine, etc.) and investigation reports. Because of the differences of the research content, and the differences of demonstration method, the paper writing form also has the differences. So strictly speaking, there is no uniform format and fixed structure. The format is a kind of writing mode explored by predecessors and used by future generations. This mode requires the paper to have eye-catching content, innovative content, scientific methods, precise arguments and rigorous and sufficient argumentation. In structure, the model requires the paper to have the title, abstract, introduction, materials and methods, results, conclusions, references, etc, so that can answer respectively the main questions.

（4）Five Basic Requirements of SCI Paper Writing

Someone summarized five basic requirements of SCI paper writing, namely 5C:

Correctness, clarity, concision, completion and consistency. A paper will not be regarded as a qualified SCI article until fulfill these 5 basic requirements.

Introduction

One of the most difficult parts of SCI articles writing is introduction (the other one is discussion). The defect of the Chinese article is that introduction is too simple to has a connotation, and does not really reflect the original research and innovation elements of the paper. SCI papers have very high requirements for introduction. A good introduction is half the success of an article. So, everyone should work hard on the introduction. To write a good introduction, the most important thing is to maintain a strong sense of hierarchy and strong logicality. These two points are closely combined, that is, a progressive relationship should be established on the basis of logicality.

1) Explain the basic content of their research field: Try to be concise and clear without being wordy, and you should aware that it is the experts in the field who are reading your paper, so use general rather than descriptive language to describe the obvious conceptions.

2) Literature review: Literature review is one of the highlights of introduction, which should be described with special emphasis. On one hand, it is necessary to comprehensively summarize the past and present situation in this field without any omission, especially the latest progress and the references to classic literature in the past (these are the two most problematic places, which should be avoided, once the reviewer points out these two problems, it probably means that you have not done enough in-depth or comprehensive work, and the negative effect is obvious). On the other hand, the literature citation and data supply must be accurate, try to avoid partial excerpts of results without reflecting the overall results of the literature, the quoted data should also be correct, especially the indirectly quoted data (that is, the data of another literature found in other literature rather than the original literature), data error will lead to a worse impression of the article! In addition, when it comes to citing literature, pay attention to prevent the impression of plagiarism, that is, it would be appropriate to summarize the description in your own expression rather than copy the original text. If the reviewer happens to be the author

of your citation, the result of copying the original text would be terrible.

3) Analyze the limitations of the past research and clarify the innovation of your own research. This is the climax of the whole introduction, so be careful.

When expounding the limitations, evaluating the previous work objectively and fairly is needed, but do not elevate the value of your own research on the basis of belittling the work of others (this is a frequent mistake in Chinese articles). SCI paper writing should never be like this. In the elaboration of their own innovation, to closely around the defects of the past research to describe, complete and clear to describe their solution. What's need to pay attention to is that do not make the topic too general, just seize a point for in-depth elaboration. As long as a solution to solve a problem wonderfully, it is a valuable article. The more innovative the description, the easier it will be captured by reviewers. Chinese articles are characterized by innovation, while English articles are characterized by the opposite, and it is excellent to solve one or two problems thoroughly and systematically.

4) Summary description of the research contents of the paper, which can be divided into different aspects to describe, to do the final finishing work for introduction. So far, writing of introduction is completed. However, after writing the introduction, it is of great importance to carefully revise and to consider whether each sentence is properly and accurately expressed.

Methods

The methods section describes the experimental

process of the paper. The writing of this process is relatively effortless, but there are many problems that need to be paid attention to. The most crucial part is the integrity and science. Completeness is the experiment in every link should be aware that does not miss some important content. The methods section can be organized according to experimental objects, experimental equipment, experimental materials, experimental records and experimental analysis methods. As long as the following four aspects can be described completely and scientifically, the writing of methods should not be the main problem.

1) Generally, the experimental objects are people, animals or some organizations, etc., their basic information should be described clearly, in addition, it should be pointed out that most foreign publications have some specific requirements on experiments involving people or animals. Some of them do not allow experimental operations on people or animals. The paper would not be reviewed or published if this rule is violated.

2) Experimental equipment. The instrument model, the manufacturer, the use of the experimental process should be described in detail. The connection between the experimental equipment should be scientific and correct and at the same time do not give people the feeling of confusion or operational error. Some steps are indispensable for the use of the device, especially for the operations that may have a specific impact on the results of the experiment. The benefit of this is to enable the corresponding analysis in the part of the discussion. For example, some equipment need to be calibrated before

use and some require recalibration after each stage of the experiment to ensure the correctness of the results. Be sure to specify your operational steps or calibration procedures so that the reviewers can analyze your results.

3) Experimental materials. Different disciplines have different requirements.

In general, it is necessary to pay attention to the necessity of material selection. In other words, it is preferable to have a certain explanation to why this material should be selected. If this point is not well described, it may cause the entire experimental process to be unsuccessful.

4) Experimental process. It is a clear description of the entire operation process of the experiment, which generally accompanied by an experimental flow chart for the explanation. There are many ways to draw a flow chart, like textual styles, the combinations of words and schematics and, so on. Separate experiments have different approaches but in general the latter is used more often (especially in experimental subjects), as it will enable the reviewer to see the experimental process at a glance. If the sketch is beautiful, you can make a good impression on the readers. Describe a clear sense of hierarchy and describe the order and association between each step clearly in order do not create an impression that the experimental process is confusing, because the reviewer ultimately determines whether your experiment is reasonable is derived from this process.

Results

Some people write results and discussion together, but most of the papers are separate, which depend on the type of the article. If your results are more appropriate to discuss at the same time with the analysis and are not suitable for analysis alone (or it is difficult to do so, and the part of the discussion becomes a chicken rib), it is appropriate to combine them, otherwise, it should be written separately.

1) Results should be informative and accurate. Accuracy means that the results must be real and cannot be forged and tampered. Informative is to provide the most comprehensive analysis results, to provide all the results obtained from the experiment to the reader, and do not deliberately conceal or omit some important results. In a sense, sufficiently informative results do not lead to the paper being rejected directly, but when the authenticity of the results is suspected, the article may be rejected.

2) Results are generally provided with tables and figures. Different magazines do not have the same requirements for the chart, which should be treated separately according to the requirements of the magazine. Generally, the perfect table shows the first-hand results obtained by the paper, which is easy for future generations to quote and compare during the research. The illustrations can show the trend of data flexibly, which are more direct and infectious. The combination of charts can complement each other and make the results more abundant. At present, people are more and more fond of providing a variety of maps, but magazines should try to limit the number of maps; because it will increase the difficulty of typesetting, the cost of the layout and the publishing house. Therefore, it is recommended that when providing the map, try

to provide the most information with the least number of maps, up to a maximum of 8. Too many pictures appear to be rosy and cumbersome, and the editor will not appreciate them. If it is vital, some forms can be replaced by tables. The image format requires different magazines, and there are many tiff formats. It is not recommended to use bmp (jpg is not available). Some people say that using vector graphics is clearer, in fact, there is no different from tiff as long as it is clear enough. Black and white pictures are free, while color pictures are definitely charged and the price is generally high.

3) When the Results and Discussion are written separately, the Results section should try not to involve comments on the results, and it is sufficient to summarize the results. Otherwise, the contents of these two parts will appear to be overlapped and cumbersome, which is not benefited for discussion. The description of the results should also pay attention to the hierarchical arrangement. It should be described separately according to the requirements of rationality, which seems to be more logical. Don't mess up and reduce the readability of the paper.

4) Results mostly contain statistical results. The form of the variance analysis should be given according to the format of the publication. Some should be provided in detail for the analysis value, degree of freedom and probability. Some can be analyzed as long as the value and probability is analyzed. Probability can be given in the form of $P = 0.02$ or $P < 0.03$, and the expression of degrees of freedom also has the special requirements.

Although these details are not really relevant, we should pay attention to the uniform of the format and do not mess with each other. When there are too many statistical analysis results, it can be expressed in the form, which can refer to the results after SPSS software analysis. If the results of the paper are all statistical analysis data, it will appear messy, but the table may avoid this situation.

Discussion

Introduction and discussion are the two most difficult parts to write. Discussion is hard to write because it is the best way to show the depth and breadth of an author's research questions. Depth is the extent to which the paper has studied the problem. The breadth refers to whether it can analyze and interpret the experimental results from multiple angles. To write a discussion, you can probably divide it into the following two steps:

1) Select the questions that you want to discuss in depth.

Some of the outcomes in the results are important, while some can be taken in one stroke. Choosing the appropriate results for an in depth discussion in the discussion section is the first question to be addressed in writing this section. Generally speaking, it can be judged according to the following principles: If your results reflect the uniqueness of the experiment and are not obtained in other studies, then the result is the problem to be discussed. Some results are consistent with previous studies, and there is no significant difference, so you should take it without having to discuss it in depth. An essential role of discussion is to highlight the innovation of its own research, and to reflect the characteristics that are significantly different from others. The important thing says there are a difference, and the difference is the innovation.

2) Selected questions should be discussed from multiple angles according to a certain level. The reasoning should have the basis and the questions should be clear and thorough. There is sometimes more than one choice (more than two in most cases), so it should be described as a certain level. In general, put the most important in the middle, and then followed one in the beginning and the end. Putting it in the middle can bring in the judge's emotions to a climax. The front is the paving, and the follow is the summary. This order seems to be more appropriate. Whether the problem is important or not, it is necessary to discuss it from multiple angles:

a. First of all, there must be a comparison of the similar results, which can indicate the uniqueness of their conclusions.

b. The secondary system explains why there are such results, and there are many methods (from the perspective of experimental design, theoretical principles, analytical methods, or other people's analytical methods, etc.). The important thing is to clarify this issue in-depth, and it is not possible to make people feel uncomfortable. (It is really difficult to do this because the reviewer always asks new questions, and we can only try to do this.)

3) Discussion section also needs to keep consistent with Results!

That is, the results and the discussion should be one-to-one. Do not indicate that the content of the discussion can lead to the opposite of the experimental conclusion, which proves that your discussion is a complete failure or your experiment is a failure. Therefore, the accuracy of the text description and language expression of the discussion is particularly important. Due to the different expressions between Chinese and English, it is necessary to avoid misunderstandings in the expression before submitting a manuscript. If the paper is rejected, it is very embarrassing.

Acknowledgments & References

Acknowledgments are divided into two main categories: the first is to indicate the source of the research fund. China is generally the Nature Science Foundation of China (NSFC, National Natural Science Foundation). The United States is mostly the National Institute of Health (NIH, National Institutes of Health). When writing a fund, you should generally mark the Grant Number. Only this can be regarded as the research result of the fund, and it can also be regarded as the research result of the laboratory. It is important to emphasize that no research results have been completed without funding. The second is to thank the participants (researchers not listed in the author) and the unit. If you pass the first trial and finally accept the publication, you will also add thanks to the editor and anonymous reviewers. This is the basic courtesy.

References are important in the format. Different magazines have different requirements for reference formats. The specific differences can be divided into:

for the author's writing method, some are shorthand in front, some are shorthand, some are abbreviated, some are short, and some of the name of the article have to be quoted, while some have no quotes; Some are written in journals, some are abbreviated, some are full, some are italic, others are not needed; Some of the order of the year and period are in the former, while some are in the post; Journal papers, books, dissertations, conference papers, and four citation formats are different; the order of the documents is in alphabetical order, while some are in Arabic of the order that they appear in the paper. Summary: Basically these questions are very trivial, but if your references are in a mess, it will make the reviewer's impression of your paper very poor. They may think that you have no cognitive organization and writing papers, resulting in certain negative impact. Therefore, although things are small but the impact is great. It is still necessary to organize them seriously. In addition, the paper should be written in English from beginning to end. Never write Chinese first and then translate it into English.

The publication of SCI technical papers should conform to the general norms of writing papers, such as the accurate use of legal measurement units, the correct use of professional terminology, symbols, abbreviations, etc., which meet the need of modern academic, information exchange and storage. In addition, depending on the type of paper, there should be a different focus on the content expression, so that the article will have distinct characteristics. For example, clinical observation and summary of efficacy should focus on the description of the efficacy, and pay attention to its comparability.

For field investigations, we should pay attention to the results of the data obtained and explore the law of the emergence and prevalence of disease, so that serving preventive health and disease prevention. For the observation class, we should focus on the difference between the measured data and the previous literature and its practical significance. For biological reaction class, the experimental data and conditions are strict, and the experimental materials and experimental conditions should be explained in detail to enhance the credibility of the results and conclusions. In addition, we also pay attention to the sample representativeness, comparability between groups, accuracy of observation results, reliability of observation indicators, accuracy of statistical processing and correctness of conclusive reasoning.

4. 投稿及修稿程序 Procedures of Manuscript Submission and Revision

（1）Submission procedure

1）Choose a journal. Combine professional knowledge, IF table and other people's experience to comprehensively select the journals to be delivered, and enter the journal query system to query the trend of articles in recent years.

2）Download introduction for submission. Just go to the home page of each magazine, open the submit paper column, click on introduction to view or download.

3）Preparation: Manuscript.doc, tables.doc, figures. tiff (jpg, etc.), cover letter, and sometimes title page, copyright agreement, conflicts of interest.

4) Submit a manuscript: First go to the home page of each magazine, open the submit paper column, first register an account as the correspondent author, then log in as author login, follow the prompts to complete: Select article type, enter title add/edit/remove authors, submit abstract, enter keywords, select classifications, enter comments, request editor, attach Files, and finally download the pdf. After checking the error, you can go to the submission page to approve the submission or directly submit it.

5) Irregular attention to manuscript status: Submit new manuscript, submissions sent back to author, incomplete submissions, submissions waiting for author's approval, submissions being processed, submissions needing revision, revisions sent back to author, incomplete submissions being revised, waiting for author's approval, revisions being processed, and declined revisions.

6) Submitted the revised manuscript: mainly modify the revised manuscript, response to the reviewers, cover letter, and other related materials. The program is to enter the main menu of the submission homepage, click revision, still deliver according to the original program, remember to modify the title, abstract and reply letter. When uploading the attachment, first check the left and unmodified material (meaning leave it unchanged), then click next, then upload the modified material (mainly including revised manuscript, response to the reviewers, cover letter, etc.) Finally download the pdf, check it is correct, you can go to the submission home page approve

submission or directly submit it.

7) Correct proof: The general editorial department first sends out three electronic documents, including query, proofs, pannotate, and sometimes paper proofs, such as a pineal research. Submit it by e-mail after proofing.

8) Copyright agreement - conflicts of interest: Usually required for the first submission, but there are a few magazines that need to be provided after accepted.

（2）Summary of submission experience

1) Choose the right SCI journal correctly. In principle, the first choice is to submit a high IF magazine, and then continue to reduce IF, but everyone knows that every time we change a magazine, we may need to change the format for a long time, unless you use document management software. Experts believe that it is not reasonable to submit a manuscript blindly. It is necessary to combine the professional knowledge.

2) It is not suitable to submit an article twice at the same time. This kind of opportunistic thing is best not to do because the editors among many magazines are the same. Once the same article is sent to the same editor or reviewer twice, the consequences are unimaginable, especially you need to transfer the agreement when you contribute manuscript, remember the main copyright issues.

3) How to correctly select the reviewers that must be recommended? General Editors will not choose the reviewers you recommend, but you should try to choose experts in your peers.

4) How to improve the success rate of a submission? The innovation of the article itself is the first factor. It is also important to choose the journal, the perfect format of the article, and the fluency of the sentence (especially in line with english habits).

5) Copyright agreements and conflict of interest forms should be carefully filled out. When signing, try not to replace the signature, so as not to be embarrassed when it is discovered by the editor.

6) Try to change the manuscript format as much as possible by referring to the submission instructions. This can measure the rigor of a researcher. It is recommended that you carefully read the introduction for submission and correct it one by one to prevent delays in peer review time.

7) After revising, you must check the corrections in the first draft: title, abstract, cover letter, etc.

8) You need to know if the journal needs to review fees and publication charges. Everyone knows that the publication charges are generally measured in US dollars. It is recommended that you choose a magazine that does not need a page fee (no color pictures is also required for the page fee). However, some magazines, such as *Endocrinology*, require a page fee. Most magazines require a page fee if they have a color picture, you should be cautious to choose.

9) The review period for foreign language SCI magazine is 1 to 3 months. Everyone waits patiently. If there is no news for about 2 months, you can check the status of the manuscript by e-mail.

5. 投稿示例 Example of Manuscript Submission

By Dr Fuling Zhou, M.D., Ph.D. from hematology department, Zhongnan hospital of Wuhan university.

Step 1: Prepare your paper, including title page, manuscript, figures, cover letter, etc.

Step 2: Choose a journal you want to publish, and open the journal homepage(Figure 4-1).

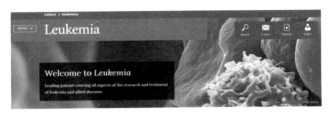

Figure 4-1

Step 3: Click "Authors" - "Author Guide" to read the contents(Figure 4-2).

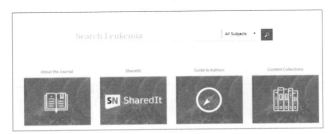

Figure 4-2

Step 4: Click "submit", then access another webpage (Figure 4-3).

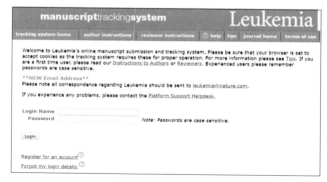

Figure 4-3

Step 5: If you are the first time to submit a paper to this journal, please click "Register for an account", then appears another webpage.

Step 6: Complete the form, click "continue" (Figure 4-4).

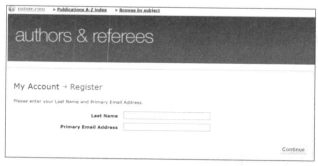

Figure 4-4

Step 7: Fill the form.

Note: The form with red* should be filled compulsorily(Figure 4-5).

Step 8: Then appear the following page(Figure 4-6).

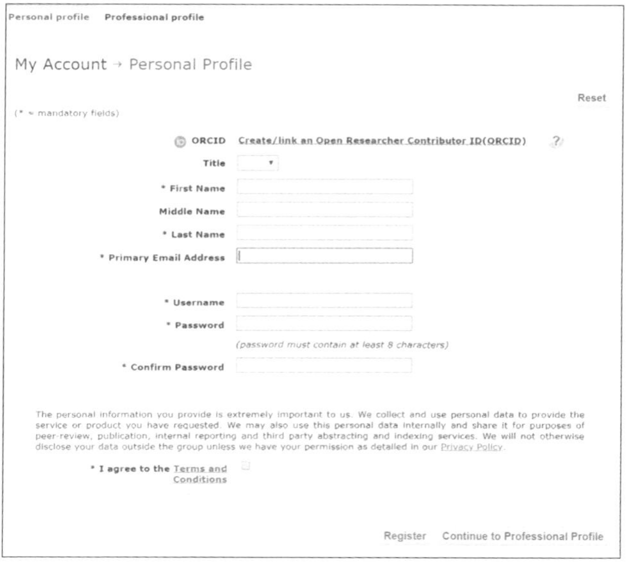

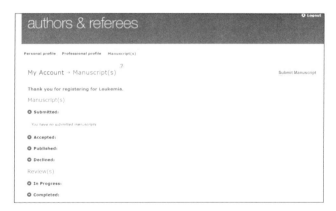

Figure 4-5

Figure 4-6

Step 9: Click "submit manuscript".

Step 10: Choose the journal you prefer(Figure 4-7).

Step 11: Click "submit manuscript" again(Figure 4-8).

Please select the journal to which you would like to submit your manuscript.

For all other journals, please click Here

```
BDJ Open
BDJ Team
Blood Cancer Journal
Bone Marrow Transplantation
Bone Research
British Dental Journal
Cancer Gene Therapy
```

Close

Figure 4-7

Please select the journal to which you would like to submit your manuscript.

For all other journals, please click Here

```
Laboratory Investigation
Leukemia
Light: Science & Applications
Microsystems & Nanoengineering
Modern Pathology
Molecular Psychiatry
NPG Asia Materials
```

Please click button to submit a manuscript to Leukemia. Submit Manuscript

Close

Figure 4-8

Step 12: Click "Article" (Figure 4-9).

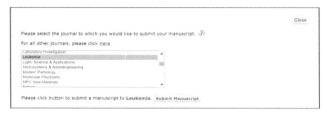

and/or change manuscript files and manuscript information by clicking on the 'Change' or 'Fix' links respectively.

4. The 'Submit' primary task is the last step in the manuscript submission process. At this stage the Manuscript Tracking System will perform a final check to ensure that all mandatory fields have been completed. Any incomplete fields will be flagged by a red arrow and highlighted by a red box. Click on the 'Fix' link to return to relevant section for completion. Once your manuscript has been finalised, click on the 'Approve Submission' button to submit your manuscript for consideration. A 'Manuscript Approved' message will display on your author desktop to confirm the submission.

Please take some time now to read the full Instructions to Authors. This will ensure your manuscript meets all Editorial requirements.
Choose the appropriate manuscript type:

- Article
- Review Article
- Editorial
- Obituary
- Comment
- Correspondence
- Perspective
- Letter

Continue

Figure 4-9

Step 13: Click "Upload files" (Figure 4-10).

Step 14: Fill the title, keywords.

Step 15: Upload all your files.

Step 16: Fill the author information and add all authors in this paper.

Step 17: Click "Approve", then submit your manuscript.

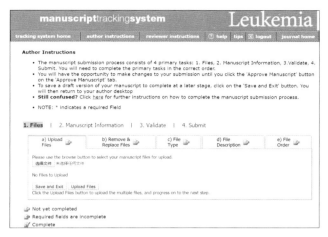

Figure 4-10

6. 医学文献阅读的策略与技巧 Reading Strategies and Tips for English Literature

For newcomers entering a field for the first time, they must read a lot of literature in order to grasp the dynamics and direction of this field. I remember a graduate student who studied in the ocean said that at first his tutor asked him to read a large number of literature, and the number was specified every day. It seems to be 100 articles. As I just came into this field, I still had no concept of many problems, which made it very difficult to read and I cannot understand many contents. I asked my mentor, only to be told to read enough each day. Later, with the increase of reading, I finally got a thorough understanding of my tutor's methods. Therefore, I think the novices should pay attention to the number of reading literature, the accumulation of more, the natural change from quantitative development to qualitative

285

change. Moreover, each author's research method somewhat has the difference. While reading, you will compare the merit and shortcomings of research methods, and this procedure will bring benefit to your own future research. In fact, due to the rapid progress of science and technology, even in your own field, there are many new technologies and new ideas emerging.So, a "veteran" will soon fall behind if he becomes lazy to update his knowledge.

When reading the literature to track the state of the art, it is important to exercise your own judgment and not follow blindly. Even well-known scientists and textbooks sometimes make mistakes. You should remember that you see the problem others will also see. The more important the problem is, and the more intensive the competition will be. If the research conditions are not as good as those of others, it is impossible for original research schemes to surpass others and achieve success without innovative research ideas. In today's plethora of literature, it feels like an increasing number of posts, without wanting to miss out on the good stuff:

(1) From point to surface. Selected questions and hot spots in the work practice, from a small branch, retrieval of more complete literature, generally the recent 20 or so has been quite a lot. Why need not care about 3 years ago, because knowledge updates very fast, and what can check on the net is the full text in recent years more. Learn how other people find and solve problems. Know the current consensus on this issue and differences. Then, expand on your interests and research goals to find out who has the most recent and illuminating articles in the field of research: Whose articles are cited the most time,

and whose articles are the most up-to-date. Go to the library and read his article in full. Gradually expand your horizons and build your own professional knowledge structure and views.

(2) From miscellaneous to essence. With a certain knowledge base, for complex literature, there should be personal judgment. Track the research progress of a topic or an expert, compare the development of arguments on the same topic, grasp the new methods or conclusions, or pay attention to the changes in the author's opinions, and explore the reasons. Cultivate personal academic accomplishment. For high quality journals, regularly browse, from the surface to understand the academic progress and hot, according to personal interests and work progress.

(3) A good memory is not better than a bad pen. Every discovery, every thought, should be written down. Case follow-up, literature review, etc. When writing articles, they are ready-made materials. Now there are computers, but writing a literature review is a good way to improve your knowledge structure. Writing down arguments and personal experience at any time, there will be twice the result with half the effort. Whether written on paper or recorded in the computer, you should have a notebook.

(4) For the downloaded literature, you should name it with its content to establish a thematic magazine according to the time of the special classification. What needs to be read carefully and saved, what is of little use, to be deleted, and what needs to be read but has not been read yet. When you think about it later, you can find it in time.

(5) Study every day. If you only work as a collector,

it loses the significance of research. The purpose of the download is to learn. Through reading, master the methods and knowledge. As long as you persist in learning, you will establish your own knowledge structure. When all else falls into place, you can do it with ease.

Reading papers is a skill to be practiced. It is impossible to read all the papers in their entirety. Reading the paper can be divided into following processes:

(1) Read the abstract for most articles and the full text for a few articles. Master a little look up through the full text, often to get the full text for fun, so there is no time to read the content of the article. Really useful full texts is not so many. Of course, it's not right to just look at the abstract.

(2) Centralize time to read the literature. Have seen will always forget. The more fragmented time you look at the literature, the more time you waste. Concentrate time to see more easily linked, form the overall impression.

(3) Record and mark: A document is copied or printed, marked or annotated directly with a pen. Documents in PDF or HTML format can be highlighted or changed in text color using the editor. This is another important way to avoid wasting time.

(4) Read the article you want to quote carefully. The misinformed caused by the cited is numerous.

(5) Pay attention to the reference value of the article. The IF of the journal and the number of citations of the article can reflect the reference value of the article. However, be aware of how other articles quoting this article to evaluate this article: Support or opposition, supplement or correction.

附录　医学英语构词法
Introduction to Medical Terminology

（1）Features of Medical Jargon

A. A vast vocabulary

B. Somewhat "peculiar" pronunciation

C. High efficiency due to word decomposability

D. Semantic deducibility

（2）Word Dissection

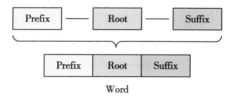

Word

Root: the determinant of semantics of a word

Prefix: adjusting the meaning

Suffix: usually helping determining the part of speech of a word

（3）Etymology

Two versions of one meaning, i.e. two roots not really worth distinguishing: Latin *vs.* Greek

e.g.

"Renal" and "nephric" both mean pertaining to the kidney.

The same root could possess diverse meanings

accordant with the context.

e.g.

myel- as in osteomyelitis (bone marrow) and myelodysplasia (spinal cord)

scler- as in sclerosis (hardening) and scleritis (sclera)

cyst- as in cystitis (bladder) and cystogastrostomy (cyst)

（4）The Concept of Combining Form

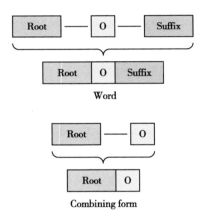

e.g.

Neur-

Neur/o-

Neurology

Neuritis

The presence of the linking "o" depends on the suffix.

（5）Suffix

1) Silent Letters and Odd Pronunciations

e.g.

dystrophy (accent on the first syllable)

euphoria (silent "e")

gnathic (silent "g")

pneumonia (silent "p")

pseudopod (silent "p")

ptosis (silent "p")

rheumatic (silent "h")

xiphoid (the weird pronunciation of "x")

2) Some Examples of Special Changing Forms

Roots ending in "x"

e.g.

Pharynx, coccyx, thorax

Their adj. forms are pharyngeal, coccygeal and thoracic, respectively.

Suffixes beginning with "rh"

hem/o + -rhage = hemorrhage (double "r")

men/o + -rhea = menorrhea (double "r")

Suffix: determinant of the part of speech of a word

Noun Suffixes, e.g.

phobia, alcoholism, acidosis

tetany, schistosomiasis, alkalosis, ketosis

dysentery, insomnia, parasitism

thrombosis, psoriasis

analgesia, sclerosis, atony

3) Physicians & Respective Disciplines

Geriatricians are doctors who specialize in geriatrics.

Podiatrists are doctors who specialize in podiatry.

Orthopedists are doctors who specialize in orthopedics.

Cardiologists are doctors who specialize in cardiology.

Nephrologists are doctors who specialize in nephrology.

Stomatologists are doctors who specialize in stomatology.

Pediatricians are doctors who specialize in pediatrics.

Psychiatrists are doctors who specialize in psychiatry.

Psychologists are doctors who specialize in psychology.

Orthodontists are doctors who specialize in orthodontics.

4) Adjective Suffixes

e.g.

cardiac, skeletal, muscular, dietary

muciform, metric, anatomical

febrile, toxoid, respiratory, venous

salivary, pelvic, neurotic, fibrous

epileptiform, ovoid, topical, virile (c.f. viral)

vocal, surgical, nuclear, circulatory

* For roots ending in "sis", adjective suffixes for them should be "-tic" in place of "sis".

e.g. psychosis, psychotic.

5) Forming Plurals

-a	-ae
-en	-ina
-ex, -yx, -ix	-ices
-is	-es
-ma	-mata
-nx (anx, inx, ynx)	-nges
-on	-a
-um	-a
-us	-i

e.g.

gingiva gingivae

foramen foramina

appendix appendices

stigma stigmata

phalanx phalanges

spermatozoon spermatozoa

ovum ova

embolus emboli

vertebra vertebrae

ganglion ganglia

omentum omenta

peritoneum peritonia

perineum perinia

testis testes

lumen lumina

matrix matrices

serum sera

meninx meninges

focus foci

pelvis pelves

adenoma adenomata

（6） Prefixes

1) Prefixes for Numbers

e.g.

monocular, unilateral, hemisphere

semiprivate, bicuspid, dimorphous

diploid, triplet, quadrant, tetrahedron

multiple, polysaccharide, quadruplet

quintuplet, quadriceps, dichotomy

fallot's tetralogy, quadruped

2) Prefixes for Colors

e.g.

Cyan/o-

Erythr/o-

Leuk/o-

Melan/o-

Xanth/p-

Chlor/o-

cyanosis, erythrocyte, leukoplakia

melanin, xanthoderma, melanocyte

xanthoma, chloroplast

3) Negative Prefixes

e.g.

aseptic, antidote, contraception

depilatory, dissect, insignificant

nonradioactive, noninfectious

unconscious, amorphous

antibody, amnesia

contralateral, incontinent

dehumidify, contraindication, antiserum

4) Prefixes for Directions

e.g.

Ab-

Ad-

Dia-

Per-

Trans-

abduct, adduct, adhere, dialysis

percutaneous, transfusion

perforate, adjacent, abnormal

transfer, transcytosis

5) Prefixes for Degree

e.g.

hyper-

hypo-

olig/o-

pan-

super-

hyperventilation, hypoxia, pandemic

oligomenorrhea, panacea

supernumerary, hyposecretion

hypertension, oligodontia

superficial, panplegia

6) Prefixes for Size and Comparison

e.g.

equilateral, euthanasia, heterosexual

homothermic, homeostatic, isograft

homograft, heterograft, xenograft

macrocyte, megabladder, megalocephaly

microscopic, neonate, neoplasm

normovolemia, orthotics, poikiloderma

pseudoplegia, regurgitation, reflux

poikilocyte, normothermic

heterogeneous, euthyroidism

isometric, megacolon, recuperate

7) Prefixes for Time and/or Position

Prefixes for Time

e.g.

antenatal, predisposition, prodrome

postmenopausal, postnasal

antecedent, projection

premature, post-traumatic stress disorder

prophase

metaphase

anaphase

telophase

interphase

Prefixes for Position

e.g.

Dextrocardia, sinistrad, ectoderm

Excise, endoscopical

Mesencephalon, synapse, telangion

Syndrome, ectocardia, synthesis

Extract, ectopic, symbiosis

Exogenous, sinistromanual

Endoderm, exhalation, inhalation, ectoparasite

（7）医学英语词根表

Prefixes

A

a- / an-

　　amenorrhea

　　(dysmenorrhea, menorrhagia)

　　auria

　　anemia

ab-

　　abnormal

　　abapical

　　abarticulation

abdomino-

　　angina abdominis

　　abdominocentesis

　　abdominouterectomy

　　abdominohysterotomy

acro-

　　acromegaly

acroarthritis (inflammation of extremity joints)

acroerythema

aden/o-

adenoma

adenocarcinoma

adipo-

adipogenesis

adiposis

adipochrome

af- (to, toward)

afferent

all/o- (different)

allopathy

allergy

ana- (up, back, again, separated)

anabiosis

anabolism

analepsia

analgesia

analgetic

analgesic

angio- (vascular - including blood vessels and lymphatics)

angiology angitis angiosis

angiopneumography

angiorrhagia angioma

angiomatosis

angiomyopathy,

angionecrosis,

angioneuralgia

angina-: acute laryngitis, sore throat

angina simplex

angina streptococcus

angina ulceromembranosus

angina pectoris (angina cordis)

angina arthritica

B

basi-/baso-

basophilia

basophil

basolateral

brachy- (short)

brachyfacial

brachydactylic

brady- (slowing)

bradycardia

(tachycardia)

broncho- (bronchu)

bronchitis

bronchial discharge, bronchopneumonia

bronchio- (bronchiole)

bronchiolitis

bronchioectasis/ectasia

bucco-(cheek)

buccobranchial

buccopharyngeal

C

cardia (heart, and cardiac portion of stomach)

cardio-

endocarditis

cardiasthma

cardiectasis

celio-

    celiocentesis

    celioparacentesis

    celiomyositis

cephalo-

    cephalocele

    cephalocentesis

cervico-

    cervical vertebrae

    cervical lymph node

    uterine cervix

chol- / chole- (bile)

    cholechrome

chloro-

    chlorosis (green sickness)

chondro-

    chondroma

choroid/o- (choroid)

    choroiditis

    choroidocyclitis

    choroidoiritis

cion- (uvula)

    cionectomy cionotomy

    colpocystocele

    colpocystitis

    colpocystoplasty

con- /col- /com- /cor- (together)

    collapse -lapse

    complex -plex

    congenital

copr/o- (feces)

copremia

copracrasia

cyano-

cyanosis

cyanopathy

D

dermato-/derma-

dermatology

dermatomyositis

dia- (across, passing thru)

diaphragm

diameter

dys- (abnormal)

dysfunction

dysmenorrhea

fibrodysplasia

myelodysplasia

E

encephalo-

encephalitis

encephalopathy

entero-

enteritis

enterectomy

enterectasis

eu- (true, good)

euphoria

eutocia

F

febri- (fever)

febrile

febrifugal

febrifuge (antipyretics)

fibro- (fibrotic tissue)

fibroma

lipofibroma

myxofibroma

fibromatosis

neurofibromatosis

fibrohemangioma

fibroosteoma

fibrosarcoma

G

gastro-

gastritis

gastrointestinal tract

glio-

glioma

gliomyxoma

glioneuroma

oligodendroglioma

glioblastoma multiforme

glioepithelioma

gravida- (pregnancy)

graviditas ampullaris

graviditas abdominalis

gravidtas intraperitonealis

gyn(o)- /gynec-/gyneco-/gyne-

gynecology

Gynecopathy

H

hamarto- (hamartia)

hamartoma

hamartoplasia

hemangio- (small blood vessels)

    hemangiectasia

    hemangioma

    hemangioendothelioma

hemi-

    hemiplegia

    hemicrania (amphicrania)

hepato-

    hepatoma

    hepatocyte

hetero-

    heteroadenoma

    heterogenesis

    heterozygote

hippo- (horse)

    hippocampus

    hippocoryza (coryza-rhinitis)

histio-

    histiocytes

    histiocytosis

    histiocytomatosis

homeo-/ homo-

    homozygotes

    (heterozygotes)

    homeochronous

    homosexuality

hydro-

    hydronephrosis

    hydrocephalus

    hydrophobia

hyper-

    hyperkeratosis

    hyperthyroidism

    hyperemia

    hypertrophy

hypo-

    hypocalcemia

    hypothyroidism

    hypofunction

    hypodermic

    hypogastric

hypno- (sleep)

    hypnoanalysis

    hypnogenic

    hypnology

K

kerato- (cornified epithelium)

    keratocyte

    hyperkeratosis

L

lipo-

    lipoma

    lipohemangioma

    liposarcoma

    lipofibrosarcoma

lympho-

    lymphoma

    lymphatics

M

mal- (defect)

    malnutrition

arterio-venous malformation

masto- (mammary gland)

    mastoplasty

mega- /megalo

    megacolon

    megakaryoblast

    megakaryocyte

menin-

    meningioma

    meningeoma

    meningiohemangioma

    meningiohemangiosarcoma

meta- (change or posterior)

    metabolism

    metanephros

myco- (branched)

    mycobacterium

myc(o)- / mycet(o)- (fungus)

    mycosis

    mycodermomycosis

myelo- (marrow, spinal cord)

    myeloblast

    osteomyelitis

    myeloma

    anterior poliomyelitis

    myeloarchitectonics

myo-

    myoepithelium

    myositis

    myoclonia

myringo- (drum membrane)

myringoscope

myringotomy

myringodectomy

myringoplasty

myringomycosis

N

nephro-

nephritis

nephrosis

nephradenoma

nephranuria

neuro-

neuroanatomy

neuralgia

neuroglia

neuroglioma

neuroblastoma

nucleo-

nucleoanalysis

nucleole (nucleolus)

nucleoliform

odonto-

odontitis

odontonecrosis

odontoma

O

odonto-

odontitis

odontonecrosis

odontoma

orchio- (testis)

orchitis

osteo-

    ostitis

    osteoma

    osteochondroma

ovi-/ovo- (egg)

    oviduct

P

pan(t)- (entire, whole)

    pangastritis

    pantalgia

para- /par- /paro- (side)

    parathyroid

    paradenitis

para- (childbirth)

    I -para (primipara)

    II -para (secondipara)

    III -para (tertipara)

    IV -para (quadripara)

    primipara

    multipara

    nullipara

    nulliparous

    nulliparity

par(a)- (neigbouring, abnormal)

    par(a)esthesia

    parosmia

    paracentral

    paracephalus

patho- / pathol-

    pathology

pathognomonic

pathodontia

pedo- (child)

pedodontia

pedodontology

pedonosology (pediatrics)

pelvis-

pelvimetry

pelviography

pelvitomy (incision of renal pelvis)

pelvioperitonitis

pelviostomy (pyelostomy)

pepsia- (digestion)

pepsin

peptonuria

peptic

per- (passing through)

perforation

peri-

perilymphatics

perifolliculitis

pero- (maimed)

perocephalus

perodactylia

peroplasia

petro- (stone)

petrosphenoid

phaco- (lens)

phacocele

phacocyst

phacitis

phacosclerosis

phago-

phagocytes

platy- (broad)

platycephaly

pneumo- (lung, respiration, air)

pneumonia

lobar pneumonia

lobular pneumonia

bronchopneumonia

pneumothorax

pneumoperitoneum

pneumocardiography

pneumopericardium

pneumohemopericardium

pneumonitis

pneumopyelogram

interstitial pnermonia

pneumocystigram

pneumorrhagia

pneumogastroscopy

pneumogram

pneumoencephalogram

pneumomediastinum

pneumocentesis

pneumococcus

polio-

poliomyelitis

poliomyelopathy

pseudo-

pseudomembrane

pseudoarthritis

pseudohypertrophy

pyel(o)- (renal pelvis)

pyelography

pyel- (renal pelvis)

pyelitis

pyelocaliectasis

pyelocystostomosis

pyelocystitis

pyelogram

pyelography

pneumopyelography

pygo- (buttock)

pygopagus

pygoteratoides

pyle- (portal vein)

pylic

pylethrombosis

pyloro- (pyloric part of stomach)

pyloroduodenitis

pylorogastrectomy

pyo- (pus, purulent)

pyocyanic

pyocyanosis

pyocytes

pyorrhea

pyocalyx

pyocele

pyopericarditis

pyoperitoneum

pyoureter

pyophthalmia

pyreto- (fever)

pyretogen

pyrogen

pyretogenesis

pyretogenetic

pyretogenic

R

ren-

renopathy

renocortical

renotrophic

renotropic

renography

renopuncture

renin

reti- (rete, network)

retiform

reticulation

reticulocytes

reticulosis

retino-

retinography

retinopathy

retinoblastoma

retro-

retroperitoneum

retropharynx

retroperitonitis

retroflexion

rheumat-

rheumatism

 rheumatic arthritis

 rheumatoid arthritis

 rheumatic fever

rhino-

 rhinitis

 rhinosclerosis

 rhinoscleroma

S

salpingo- (tube)

 salpingitis

 salpinx auditiva (eustachian tube)

 salpinx uterina (fallopian tube)

 salpingostomy

 salpingotomy

 salpingosalpingostomy

 salpingoplasty

schizo-

 schizocephalia

 schizophrenia

 schizon

spleno- (lieno-)

 splenomegaly

sterno-

 sternocostal

 sternocleidomastoideus

super- /supra-

 suprainfection

 suprarenal

sym- /syn-

 synchronia

symmetry

T

tela- (greek: tela: tissue)

telangiectasia

familial multiple telangiectasis

telo-

telomere

terato- (greek: teratos: monster)

teratoma

teratocarcinoma

teratology

teratosis

teratospermia

thrombo- (greek: thrombo-blood clot)

thrombus

thrombosis

thromboangitis

thrombopenia

thrombophlebitis

thrombokinase

tracheo-

tracheoscopy

tracheostenosis

tracheostomy

tracheostoma

tracheotomy

U

uveo- (uvea)

uveitis,

uveoplasty (uviofast)

V

vana -(vanae, veins)

  vanahemiazygos

varico-

  varicophlebitis

  varicosis

  varices

  varicotomy

  varicocele

vas- (vasa, vessels)

  vasa vasorum

  vas deferens

  vasalgia

  vasculitis

Suffixes

A

-ad (toward, to which side)

  caudad

  sinistrad

-algia (pain, algo-)

  arthralgia

  neuralgia

  myalgia

  algophobia

C

-cele (protrusion, hernia, swelling cavity)

  cystocele

  meningocele

  hydrocele

-centesis (puncture)

  dermato centesis

Cardiocentesis

E

-ectasis (expansion, dilatation)

angiectasis

bronchiectasis

-emia

anemia

septicemia

erythremia

-ectomy (excision, to cut out)

nephrectomy

Pancreaticoduodenectomy

F

-fast (resistance)

acidfast

-genesis (development, origin)

cytogenesis

glycogenesis

atherogenesis

G

-genesis (development, origin)

cytogenesis

glycogenesis

atherogenesis

-genic

allergenic

cardiogenic

photogenic

-genous

urogenous

-glossia (tongue)

macroglossia

ankyloglossia

ancylostomiasis

-graphy

Bronchography

I

-ia (condition)

anemia

algesia

analgesia

-iasis (disease)

amebiasis

ascariasis (ascarid)

schistosomiasis

urolithiasis (calculi)

-iatry (treatment)

pediatry

-itis

cellulitis

lymphadenitis

appendicitis

arthritis

bronchitis

bronchiolitis

colitis

cystitis

cholangitis

cholangiectasis

cholangiocholecystocholedochectomy

iridocyclochoroiditis

meningitis

  leptomeningitis

  glomerulonephritis

  poliomyelitis

  perineuritis

  neuritis

  polyneuritis

  panneuritis

  osteitis / ostitis

  otitis

  orchitis / testitis

L

-lepsy (seizure, sudden onset)

  psycholepsy

  epilepsy

-lith (stone)

  broncholithiasis

-lysis

  autolysis

  Hydrolysis

M

mal- (defect)

  malnutrition

  arterio-venous malformation

-malacia (abnormal softening)

  osteomalasia

  cerebromalacia

-mania

  megalomania

-metry (measurement, assay)

  Iodometry

O

-odynia (pain)

    acrodynia

-oid

    fibrinoid

    osteoid

-oma

    myoma, leiomyoma, rhabdomyoma

-osis

    cirrhosis

    erythrocytosis

    acidosis

    alkalosis

    dermatosis

-ostomy

    pancreatoduodenostomy

P

-para (childbirth)

    Ⅰ-para (primipara)

    Ⅱ-para (secondipara)

    Ⅲ-para (tertipara)

    Ⅳ-para (quadripara)

    primipara

    multipara

    nullipara

    nulliparous

    nulliparity

-parous (to produce)

    mucoparous

    multiparous

-pathy (pain or disease)

cardiomyopathy

encephalopathy

idiopathy

-penia (shortage)

leukopenia

erythropenia

-pexy (fixation)

enteropexy

gastropexy

-phage   -phagia

bacteriophages

aerophagia

-plasia (growing)

hyperplasia

hypoplasia

-plegia (paralysis)

paraplegia

-pnea (respiration)

dyspnea

apnea

-poiesis

hematopoiesis

leucopoiesis

-ptysis (coughing)

hemoptysis

R

-rrhagia (excessive discharge, esp bleeding)

hemorrhage

gastrorrhagia

enterorrhagia

-rhexis (rupture)

enterorrhexis

-rrhea (discharge)

enterorrhea

Otorrhea

S

-sarcoma (malignant tumor originated from meso- or endoderm tissue)

fibrosarcoma

neurofibrosarcoma

hemangiosarcoma

liposarcoma

endothelioma

carcinosarcoma

-static

hemostatic

hemostat (forceps)

-staxis (bleeding)

Gastrostaxis

T

-taxis (tendency, coordination)

phototaxis

-tonia (rigidity)

myotonia

-tropic

myotropy

organotropic

heliotropic

gonadotropic

(8）常用缩略语 Abbreviations

C.C.   chief complaint

H.P.I.	history of present illness
P.H.	past history
F.H.	family history
P.E.	physical examination
O.P.D.	outpatient department
E.R.	emergency room
ICU	intensive care unit
I.M.	intramuscular
I.V.	intravenous
i.v. gtt	intravenously guttae (by drip)
q.d.	quaque die
q.h.	quaque hora
q.2h.	quaque secunda hora
q.3h.	quaque tertia hora
q.4h.	quaque quarter hora
q.i.d.	quarter in die
q. suff.	quantum sufficit
b.i.d.	bis in die
P.R.N.	pro re nata
q.o.d.	quaque omni die